Why Not You?

Why Not You?

When life's experiences, circumstances, and situations reveal purpose and prepare a leader in you, then you discover your destiny.

BY DEBRA D. GIVENS

WHY NOT YOU?

November Media Publishing, Chicago IL.
Copyright © 2021 Debra D. Givens

Debra D. Givens dgivensrn@sbcglobal.net

Ordering Information: Special discounts are available on quantity purchases by corporations, associations, and others. For details, contact the publisher at the email address above.

Printed in the United States of America

Produced & Published by November Media Publishing

ISBN: 9781087978727

First Edition: August 2021

CONTENTS

A MESSAGE FROM THE AUTHOR

Life setbacks, hurts, disappointments, and unpredicted negative changes can cause one to be blinded by the bigger picture and focus on the irritants, hiccups, and bumps in the road that can cause stagnation, stand-stills, or simply put lack of motion in an individual's life. When those waves come, you may ask yourself: How do I push my life forward and become what I can see in others but not always within myself? Do I ride the wave until it settles, or do I swim on top of the wave until I get to the other side? Can I take hold of my destiny and make life what success is to me? Or, do I allow a glimpse of a faded picture to cross my mind every now and then of how things could have been? I know they say change is good, and sometimes you have to fight to get what you want. But, how do I not let fear have the position on my stage and take the major role? How do I get my fight back? What inventory of myself do I need to make to identify what life lessons I learned along the way that I may have forgotten? I want to encourage each reader to fight for themselves and never give up on you. Dismantle the picture you see if you don't like it and make a decision as well as a commitment to yourself that you will win.

Life is not made of guarantees, but it's composed of the day-by-day decisions that one chooses to make. I have learned in life to be thankful not just for the good things but also when situations, circumstances, and experiences cross your path that may not be pleasant but was needed to enhance the person that you are. They help form your character, change your outlook on life, push you to limits that you didn't know were in you, shape your very being, sharpen your knowledge, stretch your abilities, allow you to gain more self-respect, enhance wisdom, and equip you for the next life challenge with the ability to recall that you came out of that, so you'll get through this.

ACKNOWLEDGEMENTS

First and foremost, I would like to thank God for never leaving my side and giving me the ability to write this book to be an encouragement to others. It's an awesome thing to know that despite when things go left, God has a way of making them go right again. I want to thank my parents, James and Deloris Johnson, as well as my siblings Patricia Harris and James Johnson Jr, for giving me the childhood experiences that turned into some of the life lessons that equipped me for my journey. My sister has shown me how strength endures, and love can conquer any situation. I want to thank every mentor and great example that I was privileged to have in my life. Those were the individuals that stood by my side and gave me the needed tools to have the courage to make the paradigm shifts to broaden my outlook on the possibilities that, in some cases, were not easily recognized. I want to thank my amazing illustrator, Jerome Brown for capturing my vision and bringing it to fruition. I appreciate the talent, time, and detail that he put into this project to make it what I envisioned it to be. I also want to thank Tiheasha Beasley, CEO of November Media Publishing, for assisting me every step of the way. The level of commitment and quality of service was impeccable. She made the experience worth having.

SPECIAL ACKNOWLEDGEMENTS

I want to give a special thanks to my three most precious and beautiful gifts that have allowed me to have the most important title that could ever be given, MOTHER. My girls, Kourtney, Breia, and Destiny, have been my motivation as well as my inspiration. They have taught me patience, unconditional love, and the meaning of truly being a mama-bear. I want them to know that regardless of what life brings, to always seek the lesson within it, trust God, value people, have a giving heart, never give in to a give-up mindset, and conquer whatever they set their minds to do.

I want to give a special thanks to Annie Bell Givens for her consistent support and unconditional love. I know if she could speak and say how proud she was, she would. If she was able to wrap her arms around me just to remind me that she was here, she would. She always let me know that she had whatever side that I needed covered. She unapologetically cared, nurtured, and assured me that whatever I sought out to do, that would be accomplished. So, despite illness, it's the wonderful memories that remind me just how much you are still there.

I want to give a special thanks to my late aunt, Lillie Johnson. She was full of life and encouragement. She would often remind me that everything will work itself out. Losing you secondary to complications to Covid is still hard to get adjusted to, but your voice and words of encouragement will live on within me forever.

DEDICATION

Anthony Baskin (A.K.A My big brother Rick) was an inspiration, an encourager, a motivator, a giver, and had a genuine heart for people. In his eyes, there were never any big I's or little you. He highly respected everyone. He believed all were equally important and could rise to the top of any situation. His conversation included phrases such as: "What you say na," "Somebody has to do it," "Who said you can't do that?" "If you are trying to get everything you need first, what do you need faith for," "Go drive the car, walk through the house; it's not going to cost you anything," and my favorite, "Why Not You." Throughout the conversations we had, that was the phrase that always resonated within me the most. His words gave life in such a way that you believed in yourself more just because of his energy, his infectious smile, and the convincing words that he spoke with confidence and exuberance. He touched many lives. His words of encouragement will continue to motivate and live on forever in our hearts.

INTRODUCTION

When you think about where you are at this moment in your life, does it take you back to a time that only you know? The experiences, the individuals, the conversations, the mentors, the positive influences, and the negative ones that are all bottled up into one; the good, the bad, and the ugly.

I believe that there are many versions of our lives that have molded us into who we are as well as who we are evolving into. As one reads this book, my desire is for your thinking, your visions, your dreams, your expectations, and your minds to set in gear to reach a goal within yourselves that is beyond your imagination.

CHAPTER ONE

The Discovery to What Was Hidden

I grew up in Gary, Indiana with my parents, younger brother, and older sister. I am the middle child. I had days when I would think about what I would become when I grew up. My parents were not huge on education as far as pushing us to focus on a four-year degree or attending any specific college. My mother would often mention that we needed to take a trade. She would reflect on the training that she had. I can recall a picture of my mother sitting center of a class of with approximately 20 individuals in all white. It was her class picture as a certified nursing assistant, but she never worked in the field. She would mention how she would have liked to continue her education but chose to focus on raising us. Such an incredible sacrifice to make!

My siblings and I are three years apart, and as I mentioned, I am the middle child. There was a study that I read once about the "middle-child syndrome". The study suggested that the middle child is resentful, neglected, has a negative outlook on life, feels like they do not belong, is envious, least bold, and least talkative of all the siblings according to the order in which they are born. I thought this was very interesting! I wondered who the samples were, and where they came from. I know many middle children, and I just could not relate. The more I read the study, the more I was blown away. I thought to myself this may be true in some cases, but it was far from the truth for me. I was outgoing, talkative, had a positive attitude, loved to dance, and loved people. If there was a talent show, I would be the first to sign up. People would tell me that they thought I would have become a professional dancer. It was as if the music would play, and my body would know what to do. I remember breakdancing on cardboard boxes. We would flatten the boxes and place them on the ground as if it were a dance floor. It would be my brother, James (aka Boo), Tyrone, Mark, Chance, and a few other neighborhood kids. If we did not have the music, we would create our own beats. One person would beatbox while the other would rap. Beatboxing was a creative way to make sounds like drumbeats, cymbals and bass tones from a person's vocal cords without audible singing that translated into dope music. The dances ranged from the snake, wave, spins with abrupt stops with poses that were mystical yet dance poetry and whatever other combinations that were out. If there was a new dance on the scene, we were able to master it in our own way. We had moves that were out of this world. We would have block parties where the neighborhood kids were able to display their talent. It was never a question of whether I was going to participate.

I remember being in a talent show that mimicked the Gong Show with my sister Patricia at Norton Elementary School. The Gong Show was a popular talent show that aired in the late '70s. The show would have individuals who displayed all types of creative acts that people would view as talent. If the acts were not good, they would be gonged off the stage by a loud banging sound that was made by a special instrument that was hit as they were performing. When the sound was made, the contestant knew they had to leave the stage. The talent show was just that. If you were good, you were able to finish your routine, and if you were not, you were gonged off the stage. My sister and I choreographed a dance routine, of course. We would practice for hours. I was relentless. I would practice the routine with my sister and on my own. I could do the dance in my sleep. My sister attended the school. I was not a student there, but they allowed me to participate. The day of the talent show I was happy, excited, and more than ready to get the show going. Just think; me, the little sister, not only having the opportunity to go to my big sister's talent show, but I also participated in it. Dancing was in my blood and I was ready to let everyone see. We had practiced, practiced, and practiced and the time had finally arrived. The gym was full of people, and I remember my mother asking, "Are you ready?"

I responded without hesitation, "I am ready."

My sister responded, "Yes," but her face said something totally different. I looked at my sister and she had a worried look on her face. She was extremely nervous and continued to remind me of how nervous she was. She would even periodically ask me if I were nervous. I would respond, "No" and say, "Let's go over the dance again." We would practice a few steps to help stay focused. We would hear the gongs, the applause and see the acts that went before us. My mother had made our outfits. We wore powder-blue polyester bell bottom pants with a matching vest, with long-sleeve white button-down shirts with long collars. Our hair was freshly pressed, and it was styled in ponytails, one on each side. All I needed was the music, and it was about to be a dance marathon for sure – at least until the music stopped playing.

The moment had finally arrived, we were the next act. The talent before us was a modern dance that was performed by a girl named Nichole, who danced to "Black Butterfly" by Denise Williams. I can honestly say that she was awesome. As her song was fading out, the crowd applauded, screamed, and yelled out her name. I knew we had to give it all we had. They called our names; we went to the gym floor and took our positions. We danced to "I Wanna Be Your Lover" that was released in 1979 by the one and only Prince.

We started off great, and the routine was going as planned. But somewhere toward the middle my sister drew a blank. She stopped, paused, and tried to get back in sync with the music. I looked at her and saw that we were in trouble. I started freestyling, as if it was a part of the routine. I could not tell you where the new moves came from; all I know was that something had to be done quick, or we were going to get gonged off the stage. I did not want to imagine that happening. That would have been the worst. I did not take my eye off the person who was responsible for hitting the instrument that would make the devastating sound. Nor could I stop thinking about the people who were in the audience. I was determined not to be like the act that was gonged and was crying behind the stage. I said to myself, "There has been way too much work put into this dance to get gonged." I kept smiling and thinking *Who would gong a kid?* Somewhere within the course of the song we got back in sync with each other. We had changed an entire segment of the routine.

Well, we did not get gonged, and we were able to finish. However, we did not win the talent show; the girl that danced to "Black Butterfly" did, and she deserved it. But I discovered that I had the ability to think fast on my feet, keep moving (literally) and not let them see me sweat. I did not see it then, but little did I know the shaping of life was occurring. I have come to realize that the molding process of who I was becoming had started way before I had the wisdom to know it. The leader in me was being tapped into and I did not have the ability or knowledge to recognize it at that time. Life has a way of giving lessons and developing our character despite the recognition of the moment in time.

I must admit that even though I loved to dance, I also loved to climb trees, jump off roof tops, pop wheelies on my bike and jump out of swings. Whatever the boys could do, I believed I could do it even better. I played baseball and I must admit that I played it well. When I tried out for the team it taught me not to be afraid to stand alone despite what others may think. I was the only girl in the entire league of Ambridge who tried out. Of course, the boys and some of the coaches had a problem with it until they noticed my game, meaning the way I played. I had to show them that a girl could play just as well as a boy, despite what popular opinions may have been. Little did they know that I was even more determined to make the team because of the negative energy I received about trying out. I had only played baseball with the neighborhood kids. Some of the players who were trying out were not strangers to baseball because they had previously played on the league. I did not let that intimidate me even though I was nervous. I believe the thought of them not wanting a girl in the league made me mad enough not to think about how nervous I was.

I did it, I made it for one of the teams. This was one of the newer teams in the league and the coach was willing to take a chance on me. Our uniforms were brown, yellow, and white. I was excited! My coach was not concerned about me being a girl and he did not give me any slack. He pushed me just as hard as he pushed the boys. What I eventually learned was that most of my team members were new to the league. We would practice, and the more we did, it became clearer and clearer that we needed to practice even more. I can laugh about it now, but it was serious business for me then. I had some team members who wanted to catch everything coming, others were afraid of the ball and a few played the game well.

My brother, James (aka Boo), played right beside me, he was on the team as well. When it was time to play, I would have my baseball hat on, a wad of gum in my mouth, and cleats on my feet. I played center. I was not afraid of the ball and my speed was pretty good. I could throw the ball just as quick as I caught it. I often felt like the watchman on the team. I had to gauge the hit of each ball and was quick to call out, "I got it," when I saw a ball headed my way. The coaches and boys from the other teams started to notice how I played. I must admit we did not win a lot of games, but the other coaches wanted me to leave the team I was on and switch to their team. I did know that their teams were more developed and were winning. I hated to lose! My coach was aware that some of the other coaches were approaching me to join their team. At one point we were on such a losing streak that my sister would call us "The Bad News Bears." Talking about sisterly love and encouragement! Deep down inside that is how I felt at times. Regardless of the immediate gratification I would have received from being on a winning team, I had a loyalty to my coach and the other players.

There is a saying: "The grass may look green on the other side until you have to cut it." I was too young to understand the value of not being quick to move based on what is not happening, but the principle was still practiced. It was clear that in some situations some things are innately in an individual. I have come to the conclusion that when decisions need to be made, there are questions one can ask. How can I make the situation better? Am I making moves based on my emotions? Have I counted the cost if I choose to make a move and things do not work as planned? Is fear and familiar territory causing me to stay stagnant? Looking back on that situation, I would have made the same decision. Ask yourself, "Can I make a sound decision to stay or leave regardless of what the situation may be – a relationship, a job, or a location change – and know that it was the best decision that worked for me?" Never make an emotional decision and always take the time to count the cost. The decisions one makes are a direct reflection on where one is in one's life at that moment. Deciding to stay with my team despite the lack of wins was not easy. My mother was also approached by the other coaches and it was clear that we were on the same page. We supported the team who gave me a chance and not the ones who could not see my value until after they observed my skills.

I went from always wanting to dance to playing baseball, hanging with neighborhood friends, even having a club with girls from the block, Esther, Toya, and a few others. We would draw poster-size pictures and sell them for 25 cents, help the older neighbors carry their groceries in the house and do light chores for them. Despite the small token that my neighbors would occasionally give, the act of helping others was the greater lesson. Doing for others would do something within me. I gave what I was able to make the load lighter for someone else. I desired to do even more and would often think how I would like to support others when I had greater means to do so. I learned that it is a gift to give and do for others, especially without expecting anything in return. I was always willing to lend a helping hand and always desired to do more. I knew one day that desire would become a reality. I did not know for who or when, but it was something that I held on to.

I reached the point when I desired to work and have more responsibilities, with the idea of having an income, even though it was not going to be much. I was approximately 14 years old. My family would at times gather in the living room and watch television and have small family talks. My father is a pretty good jokester. He could have you laughing so hard that tears would come out of your eyes. He would tell the jokes, or you were maybe the joke. My mother is more serious and would sometimes say without a smile on her face, "James, you play too much." As we were having one of those nights, I asked if I could have a paper route.

The room got quiet, and my dad said, "That means you would have to get up to deliver the papers on time."

I understood what I was asking for because I was clear as to what I wanted to do. So, I thought! I was determined to deliver those papers as if I were making a million dollars, and I did just that! Rain, sleet, or snow, I made sure my papers were delivered on time. The one thing I did not like was collecting payments. It was a hassle. The same individuals every week had an excuse as to why they could not pay their bill on time. That would mean that I would have to make an additional trip to their homes. Sometimes the date they gave me to return would change. After several months I concluded that this was not working for me. I decided to quit. I celebrated by taking my friends from the neighborhood to McDonalds.

It was not too many months afterwards that I turned 15 years old. I still desired to work, but was not old enough to get any employment other than delivering papers. That was not an option for me anymore. I went to Kentucky Fried Chicken and spoke to the manager about employment. I knew I was not old enough, but I figured a conversation could not hurt. We hit it off well. She saw that I was determined, energetic, enthusiastic, and prepared to put my best foot forward. She told me, "If you got a work permit you are hired." First thing that next morning I was en route to get a work permit. I filled out the required paperwork and thought to myself, *KFC here I come.*

I could not believe that I actually had to go to a training that lasted a few days that was set up like a classroom to put chicken in a box. The training was not at the location where I was going to be working, it was at a corporate office. I was amazed at how serious and intense the training was. I had a moment when I was scared that I was not going to pass the chicken test. There was an actual test where you had to properly pick out the parts of the chicken, name them, identify if they were white or dark meat, and a few other things. I would not have imagined that I would be stressing over chicken. The training was well organized. I was shocked at how well versed they were with the history and the goal of the organization. I gained a new respect for KFC after taking the training. I had never experienced anything like that before.

I took my KFC job seriously. You would have thought I had stock in the company. My training continued when I was in the store. Wherever she assigned me, that is where I went. I never complained or caused any trouble. She worked with my school schedule and would occasionally have me on the late shift. One day shortly after the store opened two men came in and were very cordial. They ordered a two-piece meal and a pop. I was scheduled to work the front register. They sat in the dining area and shared a piece a chicken and asked for an additional cup. It was normally slow when the store opened, and traffic picked up later in the day. I initially felt strange when they walked in but brushed it off as nothing. One of the men would look out at the window and the other man was gazing at the front of the store. After they finished eating, they left. I went out and cleaned the area. They did this for a few days.

Several weeks went by and I noticed a male quickly go to the restroom when he entered the door. Something about him looked familiar, but I could not recall because I did not get a very good look at him. Shortly afterwards he came out of the bathroom with a ski mask running toward me pointing a gun and demanding, "Give me all the money from the register." Immediately, the voiced sounded familiar, but I was in shock. I had never had a gun pointed at me in my life. I never called out to anyone, I could hear my co-worker talking and laughing loudly in the back. I was waiting on more chicken to come out just before he demanded the money. Ironically, the cook never came from the back with the chicken, the phone did not ring, no one came into the store or the drive thru. It happened so fast. I was giving him the loose change, bills, paper clips whatever just to get him out of the store. When he left I felt relieved, thankful and blessed. You never know: one distraction, big or small, could have cost me my life, or someone else's.

I let out a piercing scream, "I've been robbed!" I was scared, nervous, pissed and shook up all at the same time. The more I thought about the voice, the more it sounded like one of the guys who would come in the restaurant when we would first open or an employee who had been terminated months prior. I was positive of this, that one out of the two of those men were the one that pointed that gun at me. The person who robbed the store was never caught, but to this day I know the familiar voice but cannot pinpoint the mystery person behind it. I did not last there long after that. Working for KFC was never the same after that experience. The writing was on the wall, and even though my manager begged me to stay, it was time for me to hang up my chicken wings and fly away.

Several months later I went to work at the neighborhood grocery store, Value Mart. I worked the register and when we were slow, I would put up the overstocked items. I felt like I had finally found a job while in high school that was the perfect fit. The managers were good people. Mr. O'Neal was the best. He was laid back but at the same time expected you to do your job. He had a bushy curl, wore glasses and was on the mid-heavy side. He would give us nuggets of wisdom every now and then on life-making decisions, finishing school and whatever else he deemed as being important. He was a state-of-the-art type of boss that let us know that he had our best interest at heart. The other manager, Mr. Gordon, was tall and slim with a mustache and a short haircut. He would walk around the store and do his checks and balances. He would try to be stern many times but let his sarcastic nature come out. He would crack jokes and go right back to trying to be serious. It was hilarious to watch. He was a good manager as well. Their styles were different, but they both desired the same, and that was that we make something out of ourselves.

The cool thing I liked about it was several kids from school worked there as well. It was almost like I never left school. There was Damon, Tommy, and of course, I could never forget Jamel. He would stock and occasionally bag groceries. He was one of the baseball team members that would tease me years prior because I was a girl playing ball. When we were at work, regardless of what the conversation was, he would try to get a joke in. In the back of my head, it was already programmed to say, "Ok, here we go." His number one throw-back moment was always, "I remember when I saw you on the field, you was all dirty and stuff. You were the only girl out there trying to play ball. Y'all never won a game. That is why you should have been on the winning team. Of course, you didn't know no better." I got to the point that I would just let him talk. There was only so many times that the facts could be set straight. It was not rocket science. Of course I would be dirty, sweaty and everything else if I am playing on a team, on a hot field, constantly moving, running bases, working the field, swinging a bat, etc., etc., etc. I was a key player, not a bench watcher. I had to remind him that, yes, we did win some games – now it may not have been many, but there were a few. The main reminder was that even though, yes, I was a girl, it was awfully strange that his coach wanted to draft me. Usually once I made that point, he would quiet down. I think the Mars vs Venus (Male vs Female) theory may have some validity. I remember many days putting my hand on my forehead and thinking, *Boy, oh boy, oh boy. What a charmer!*

The other schoolmates that I worked with were always positive. They were good, down to earth people that made working there that much more enjoyable. Tommy was quiet and never had anything negative to say about anyone, even in a joking manner. He would smile, speak, and engage in small talk every now and then. Damon would often joke lightly and laugh, but was always pleasant. He always knew when to separate conversations and joking time from being productive. It was a good team. There were a few other kids from school who worked there but they did not stay long. Working and going to school was not unusual for me, but it meant that I had to be responsible to get the grades and balance a work schedule, which I did without giving it much thought. I realized my work ethics were developing the moment I said, "I do" to employment. I worked there throughout my high school year. I would often think to myself that I had been working since I was 14 years old. Within that time span I had so many discoveries within myself that were hidden until the right situation, experience or exposure presented itself and pulled it out of me. Little did I know that life was just beginning, and I was being groomed for leadership and even greater responsibilities that I never saw coming.

Life Lesson

Never turn your back on an individual who
has believed and stood by you for people
who recognized your gifts, talents, and
abilities after you were given the platform.

What are some of your fondest childhood memories?

____

____

____

____

What valuable lessons were attached to some of your child-hood memories?

____

____

____

____

Think of one thing you decided to stay in, despite there not being many victories. Explain why you stayed.

____

____

____

____

Have you ever had a frightening experience that caused you to see things from a different perspective? If yes, what was it and what views changed.

CHAPTER TWO

The Moment of Impact

I honestly thought I was going to be a hairdresser. I have my dad to thank for that. You see, during my first year at the Gary Area Career Center it was required that you selected a field that you were interested in. I enrolled in cosmetology. The course required that you purchase a kit that cost 100 dollars. I could picture the curlers in my hand and making hair magic happen in my chair. I recalled being excited and telling my dad that I needed the money to enroll in the class. He looked at me and without a thought said, "You need to find something that's free." I recalled saying, "Dang, I know he has the money, he's just being cheap." I was upset because this is what I thought I wanted to do. It is amazing how life has a way of moving in directions that you never saw coming.

So, after hours of reviewing the classes I could enroll in, I settled for the nurse aide course. I can honestly say at the time I was not interested in nursing. That is why I often say, "Nursing found me; I didn't find it." I did not want to be at school all day. Let me explain. The Career Center is an educational institution that allows juniors and seniors to attend a half day and go to their respective schools the other half. The Career Center is designed to give each student that attends the fundamental foundation that is needed with a legitimate certificate, skills, and abilities to enter the workforce after high school. It was a great program that gave me and others another perspective and an opportunity to determine their career path. I can remember when I did my first rotation in clinicals. I was assisting a nurse who was doing wound care by holding the resident on his side. I had never seen a wound of any kind and this was my first time touching another individual to provide care. The resident did not have a backside – his buttock was completely gone. As the nurse proceeded to remove the gauze and the tape, I can recall telling the nurse and my instructor that I had to go to the restroom. My head was spinning, my heart was palpitating, I was extremely hot, I could not breathe. I felt nauseated, queasy, and lightheaded. While in the restroom I splashed a copious amount of water on my face and took multiple deep breaths. I laid on the floor until all the symptoms subsided. It felt like I was lying on the floor for hours. I will never forget that moment. My instructor knocked on the door and asked me if I was okay. When I answered, "Yes," she walked away and never questioned me. I believe she knew exactly what I was dealing with and let me have that moment to get myself together. I will never forget how uncomfortable, nervous, sick, and fearful I felt. I had no idea how the body could break down and develop open areas that one could literally put their entire hand in.

I was enrolled in this program for two years. During my junior year I would attend high school in the mornings and would go to the Career Center in the afternoons. For my senior year it switched, and I attended the Career Center in the mornings and high school in the afternoons. As time went on, I noticed myself becoming more comfortable with my skills and the material that I learned. I can recall making my first bed, taking my first set of vitals, reading a thermometer for the first time as well as passing my skills and written test. I had no idea what was waiting ahead. Despite the knowledge and skills that I gained, I did not have the mental capacity to have a clear understanding of the magnitude of the field I was training in. Boy, did I have an awakening! I thought it was an awesome thing that by default I was launched in a field that I grew to like, all because my dad would not buy a hair kit. It is amazing how life works! I had no idea of the journey that I was about to experience. I could not have foreseen what was waiting for me on the other side. Just imagine a path that started as a disappointment that grew into a like, developed into a love and ended as being my passion.

When life makes a turn in a direction that you did not foresee or plan it is possible that the intended target could have been redirected because your aim was off.

Redirected

My first job was in a long-term care setting. It was my first job as a health care provider. I can recall being nervous and excited. I had worked at other places – the neighborhood grocery store, Kentucky Fried Chicken and a newspaper route – and I can recall feeling the same way, but this time it was completely different. For the first time in my life my role was to take the compassion that I had for people and care for individuals that relied on me to assist them to make their life experience better because of my touch. I took it very personal. Regardless of where I was assigned, I wanted my personal signature, quality at its best, on the work that I did. I wanted my residents to look their best, smell their best and feel their best, I took pride in the work that I did. Just think: I was fresh out of high school and I was a certified nursing assistant! I was proud of my accomplishment. I felt great knowing that my job was helping others. I did not take it lightly. To me, this was serious business.

I remember one of my nurses pulling me to the side because I had several family complaints. If you can recall, I mentioned my original plan was to be a cosmetologist. Well, within my first few months I worked in a unit called the Atrium. This unit had mostly Caucasian residents. Because I wanted my residents to look good, smell good etc., etc., etc. I would always bring extra supplies to work, such as perfumes, powder, hair bows, Vaseline, lotions etc. So, I would use Vaseline as grease on the resident's hair and slick it down. I would wrap their hair around their heads to give them a popular hairstyle at that time called a wrap. I soon discovered that some of the families wanted to wrap me alright. Since I never attended a class in cosmetology, I did not realize that grease, especially Vaseline, was not and should not have been used in hair, especially Caucasian residents' hair. I can laugh about it now, but it was not funny at all during that time. I felt terrible. It was not my intention to get anyone upset and I had never had a family member complain about me. I was devastated!

After I was informed of the complaints by my supervisor, I immediately went into problem-solving mode. I worked the day shift and I wanted to correct the concerns with the families. I decided to pick up a shift, which meant I was going to work a double. The goal was for me to meet the families face-to-face and apologize for my error. I also gave each resident a shower to remove the grease from their hair. I was not asked to speak to the families or give showers. I did not let anyone in on the plan. I was not sure how my supervisor would have felt about me speaking to the families. As the families came in during the evening shift to see their loved ones, one by one, I revealed to them that I was the one responsible for the shining, slicked down hairstyles that they complained about. Initially I felt very uncomfortable and nervous, because I did not know how they would respond or if my supervisor would find out and have an issue with me for speaking with them. I explained to them why I decided to work a double and that I honestly did not mean any harm. They were pleased to see that all the grease had been removed from their loved one's hair and thanked me for apologizing to them. To my satisfaction, my goal was accomplished. I was tired yet determined to let every family member know personally just how sorry I was and that it would never happen again. I could have chosen not to take responsibility for my action and displayed a totally different attitude, but in the long run it would have only hurt me.

Having the ability of knowing when to humble yourself is a choice that anyone can choose to make. I say this because criticism or correction is not always taken well. Some individuals do not want to be corrected regardless of how large or small the concerns are. They do not want anyone to say anything to them even when it is needed. It is one thing to not want to be corrected, or to refuse to hear constructive criticism or guidance. It is another to be outspoken with a bad attitude, be disrespectful or have an uncontrollable temper because one feels that one has justifiable reasons as to what was done, regardless of whether it was wrong and they felt that it was the right thing to do. I believe that the root cause of not being able to hear constructive criticism or take heed of guidance, especially when it is coming from a healthy place, is pride.

Pride indeed does come before the fall. In many cases pride has set in and formed an alliance with an individual and has tricked them to believe that they are *always* right, regardless of what the facts may show or what is brought to them from the individual who has authority over them. I do not think pride in every case is the only emotional hindrance, because there can be many more that travel together, but it is truly one of the heavy hitters. Other areas that may need to be addressed are hidden jealousies, resentment, rejections, and low self-esteem, just to name a few. I am one who knows that correction, constructive criticism and having to follow guidance is not always easy, but it is necessary to get you to a place of maturity and elevate you to your next level in life. Just think: no one likes to be called into the principal's office and given a negative report about themselves. It is human nature! The bottom line is that if someone in authority corrects you, be humble enough to listen, take everything in that is being said, meditate on it, reason with yourself as to how things could have been done differently, decide to receive what was said, make the changes needed, then be patient and help someone else along the way. If your emotional state is something you cannot control due to another issue, get the help you need so your life can progress in the right direction. Seeking professional help can be the answer to the new you. The saying is true: your attitude can determine your altitude. I can say that as a result of my actions the families were very thankful, and I remember feeling like I turned a non-intended concern and negative emotional feelings into a positive outcome.

Life Lesson

Just because your intent is good, and
your motives are pure, it does not mean
it is the right thing to do or that it will be
received well by the one you are doing
it for. Taking responsibility is not always
easy, but it is always necessary.

List areas in your life that you did not plan but things worked in your favor:

____

____

____

____

What were some key areas that needed to be corrected, but criticism and direction was difficult to receive?

____

____

____

____

Give three reasons as to why it was difficult:

____

____

____

Name areas where constructive criticism, guidance and correction have given you the jump needed to push you to a better you:

____

____

____

____

Don't Rush the Process

I think that it is safe for me to say that in life we all have moments, situations, circumstances, or experiences, if not all, that we will never forget. It does not matter how much time goes by or how old we get, there are some things we can visualize and play over and over in our minds as if it occurred only moments ago. This is a good thing if it causes you to measure your growth, reflect on your level of maturity, think about the advancements you have made in life or reminisce on the lessons that were taught by those who are no longer here with you. I do understand that not all memories are positive, but it is up to the individual to decide if they will allow themselves to be hindered or stagnated, and not move past the negativity that has occurred in their life.

I know a very wise pastor by the name of Charles Jones who would say, "You cannot un-spill spilled milk," meaning that what has happened has happened. The rebound effects of an occurrence may not be easy to overcome, but it is possible. How do you turn a negative into a positive? How do you prevent what has happened to you from happening within you? How do you make the best out of a bad situation? Know that there will be a process you will have to trust in.

"Process" means a series of actions or steps taken to achieve a successful outcome. The steps can be small but meaningful. To have the ability to recognize and acknowledge the hurt is the first step of healing. Ignoring or choosing not to confront an issue can be dangerous and show up in the room in other ways. Bring God into the equation and know what he says about you: that you are an overcomer, the apple of his eye, precious in his sight and more than a conqueror. Seek therapy to walk you through areas that need to be uprooted and destroyed. Lastly, seek to forgive so that you are not hindering the progressive moves in your life that you have been destined to make. I often say, "One day at a time." Do not rush it or give up on the process, because it is only when you give up that you rob yourself of the greater you that is to come.

Life Lesson

Getting where you want to be may mean
you have to acknowledge areas that you
may want to stay dormant or buried.
To confront and address issues can be
painful, scary, and upsetting, but the
outcomes are rewarding, renewing and
progressive. You cannot un-spill spilled
milk, but know that it does evaporate,
and it can be wiped up.

CHAPTER THREE

God Does Not Make Mistakes

I do not believe my place of employment was chosen by co-incidence. I experienced a major turning point in my life. I will never forget it. Throughout my career it has been a place I go back to reflect on. It is a memory that sits on the apex of my heart. I had no idea that when I walked into that facility my life would never be the same and it would change my outlook, my views and thoughts concerning what I was purposed to do. As I mentioned, when I started as a certified nursing assistant, I worked on a unit called the Atrium. I was there for several months before I was moved to other units. The Atrium was in the basement of the facility and there were five floors. The higher the floor, the more care the residents needed. I was mainly between the second and third floor. Mamie, Clarence, Shirley, Tracy, and Joslyn were some of the aides that I worked with. They were amazing. They put the "T" in teamwork. There was never a time that if I needed them, they were not available to help me out. If anyone was going on break or needed to leave the unit for any reason, it was not an issue as to who was going to cover their side. Covering our unit was not a problem.

The nurses would make the assignments and give us reports. I was always the one who was adamant about getting a report before starting my assignment. I had witnessed major hiccups from the lack of communication between the nurse and the aide. Let me explain. I can recall a resident who was scheduled to have several labs and a diagnostic test done. He had an order to be NPO (nothing by mouth) after midnight. The resident had already missed a previous appointment and his family made arrangements to accompany him on this one. They wanted to make sure he made it to the appointment as scheduled. There were two nurses who worked on the morning of the appointment. The nurse who was responsible for my side gave the aides the report because she knew I was not going to get started until I was given a report. I always felt that it was important to have the aides come together for report so everyone could hear what was needed just in case someone needed to cover a side that they were not originally assigned. The second nurse who was assigned to the unit was giving out medication to the patients and never came to the stations to give report. Despite me advising the aides to get report, they decided to start their assignments without it. Also, a sign was never placed on the door to indicate that the resident was NPO. During that time posting a sign on a patient's door was not a violation of there privacy, and it did not violate any hospital policies—though today healthcare agencies take extra precautions to protect patient's confidentiality. So that morning, the breakfast trays came up and I am sure you can guess what happened. Yes, the resident received the tray, and he ate everything on it. The family arrived shortly afterward, and they were furiously demanding answers. Immediately there was chaos. Then the blame game started. The nurse said she informed the aide. The aide said the nurse never gave her report. Dietary claimed they never got a slip. There were some major screw-ups that caused a resident to not get a diagnosis or be treated timely, the facility lost a patient, and several employees were disciplined, with two ending in a termination. If only communication, documentation, follow-up and follow-through were a priority. It was amazing how people get amnesia when things hit the fan. I can say that this was not a frequent occurrence, but it was one of those experiences that was involved in my developing stages.

Like any industry, there are some positive work ethics you may witness and there are some negative ones. There were some good nurses and there were others who I had to question, not necessarily their knowledge but their professionalism. There was one nurse who was extremely lazy. She would buy a family meal of Kentucky Fried Chicken and eat it throughout the shift at the nurse station. If I was busy in a room with a resident, she would yell down the halls for me to answer patient calls while she went back to the nurse station and ate. I could not understand why she could not answer the call or why she was eating at a dirty nursing station. It would frustrate me when we would be short staffed and my name was consistently being called to answer patient call while the nurse would be eating, laughing and on personal calls enjoying the *working* hours. Just think, she was getting paid to work in a professional setting and had a fully laid out smorgasbord at a nursing station, which was one of the first things you would see when you get off the elevator. Whenever I would see her doing that it would irk my soul. I could just scream every time I would see it. I got to the point that I had to say something. I remember having a conversation with the nurse and it went in one ear and out the other. It was a total waste and afterwards she had the audacity to write me up for a bogus reason. It never made it to the front office. Remember, at this time I was not a nurse, but it did not take heaven to fall from the sky to know that this type of representation for such an honorable profession can send the wrong message. It just did not sit well with me when family members needed to speak to her and they saw bones, leftover dried mashed potatoes and the cob from the corn resting on the desk while asking for updates concerning their family members. Her behavior was eventually addressed. I remember wondering, *What took you all so long?* To this day I have a strong pet peeve with nurses eating at the nursing station. It is amazing how your experiences can stick with you in such a way that you can either adapt to it or vow to never be like it. I thanked her for the example I knew not to set.

Life Lesson

Be careful not to become the negative
example that someone sees.

What are some situations, circumstances, or memories you have that you can say have helped to shape you to a better you?

____

____

____

____

If you have experienced any negative situations, what have you done to not allow them to hinder you from moving forward in life?

____

____

____

____

Have you ever been involved in a situation where the lack of follow-up and follow-through caused a major issue, and the blame game began? What could have been done to make a difference?

____

____

____

____

What have you witnessed that did not represent the job or profession that the individual was representing? What was your immediate thought?

____

____

____

____

No Excuses

The one thing about healthcare is that it comes with its own share of challenges. During this phase of my journey a shortage of staff was the challenge. Of course, in moments like this you assist as needed and work where you were asked to cover. Initially there were only certain floors and specific residents that I would be assigned to. But like the times, things change. The idea for me to be able to work where I was assigned allowed me to embrace the word "flexibility". I never complained because my thoughts were, if I punched the clock, they had the responsibility of scheduling me for the hours I agreed to work. I had been to numerous in-services and was very clear on the meaning of continuity of care. The goal, like any other institution, is to have individuals that were equipped, confident in their role with good people skills and ultimately can perform the care as well as the routinely scheduled employee would do. Yes, continuity is always best, but flexibility can be even better if individuals have the mindset that if care is what is needed, they have the tools and the ability to make it happen.

Of course, goals are set, but not always reached. I cannot speak for everyone else, but I can say when I had a new assignment, I tried my best to find out as much about that individual as possible. I would introduce myself and let them know I was going to be caring for them for the remainder of the day. In one of those instances when I was given an assignment for the first time on a floor that I never had, I remember caring for a very small-framed female in her 70s. She required total care, which means she relied on someone to perform ADLs (activities of daily living) for her. I would describe her as being someone who was stuck in time. It was clear she was raised in an era that she related to. She would turn on her call light and expect you to be there within seconds.

On this day she had multiple family members in her room to celebrate her birthday. I was called in the room to clean her up because she was scheduled to go out of the facility with her family. She wanted to stay in the bed until they arrived. As I entered the room, I greeted everyone with a smile and asked how everyone was doing. I was already pre-warned by my nurse of the behavior that she would display. I had another aide accompany me, as had been advised. As I went to say happy birthday, she immediately stated that she needed to be cleaned. I was thinking to myself, *Ok, so far so good.* I thought maybe because she had a large amount of family members and I was being friendly she would be just fine today, meaning no behaviors. I was sadly mistaken. She looked at me and turned toward her family members and yelled out loudly several times, "Oh they love to wipe my ass, that's what they do best." Her entire family turned beet red with embarrassment. All of them began to apologize, and some of them where in tears. I was not shocked, because I had been warned about this kind of thing, so I had prepared for much more than what she said. I asked the family to step out of the room and had the nurse speak with them after I reassured them that I was ok and there was no need for them to be upset over what had been said. I had to take a moment, because that was the first experience of that kind that I had ever had. I proceeded to complete the task and got her ready so she could go out and enjoy her family. I spoke to several of my colleagues about my experience, and I stopped complaining after I heard their encounters with her.

During our down times, my co-workers and I would sit in an area on the units where there were chairs and a couch or two. In that room was where I would hear about all the news that was floating in the facility. On one day I was informed of a new resident who was recently admitted. She was known as "the young black girl who was admitted to the fifth floor". I was told she was admitted approximately three weeks prior. They did not know her name, but they told me that she had an aneurysm while giving birth. I told them about a friend of mine who I grew up with who had a similar story. I stayed several blocks from her, and we went to elementary school together. I would see her when I would visit my best friend, who stayed across the tracks from her. When we were in high school, we lost contact. One of my neighbors who lived three houses down from me told me that she was pregnant. I could not believe it! I saw her several times while she was pregnant, and she would tell me that she was excited and scared at the same time. She told me that she would have to take something for an occasional headache but other than that she was okay. Several years went by and I completely lost contact with her, but I saw one of her relatives and she informed me that she had the baby and experienced an aneurysm while giving birth. I was devastated, confused, hurt, and deeply saddened. She had lived but was in a vegetative state. I reminded myself often after hearing that just how quickly things could happen. As I told the story, my curiosity grew stronger as to who this person on the fifth floor was. I was clear I did not want to see her or take care of her, because one of my colleagues had already mentioned to me that she was one year younger than me.

I could barely work, seeing that I had already had a day that I would never forget, but it got even worse. The supervisor who was scheduled on this day was the very one that I would try to avoid as much as possible. She was very tall, with bushy salt and pepper hair, stoutly built, with a strong voice. I was told that she was mean and unapproachable and would only speak once in a blue moon. I was so bothered by what I was told that I could not leave without knowing the name of the mysterious resident that was admitted on the fifth floor. I gathered my fears, took a deep breath, and walked up to her as she was making rounds on my unit. I politely asked if I could speak with her for a minute. She was in a very good mood and replied, "Yes, you may." I was shocked! I proceeded to ask her about the new resident who was recently admitted on the fifth floor. She did not go into detail, but she gave me her name. I was sick and had to leave for the day. It was the name that I suspected but was praying not to hear. I was crushed, my head was spinning out of control, I felt like I needed to throw up, I was weak and could not stop crying. This was so devastating! I was so unprepared for what would happen next. I took two days off so I could get myself together. This newly found information laid very heavy on my heart and caused me to change the way I look at life.

I went to work saddened that she had to be there, that her life as I once knew it was a memory of the past. This was my first experience knowing a person my age that was in a nursing home and required total care. Remember, there was a shortage, and coverage of the units was needed, regardless of whether you had a permanent assignment. My previous interaction with my supervisor was quite pleasant, so I went to her again and explained my situation. I informed her of the relationship that I had with the newly admitted resident. I let her know about the friendship we had with each other. I pleaded with her not to assign me to that unit because I could not imagine caring for someone who I had such a close relationship with. There were many days that I would say to myself, "This is too much," but something on the inside kept me going. If I was not assigned to the fifth floor, I was okay. To my surprise, my supervisor did everything she could to assist me. That was the moment that I realized not to listen to the experience of others as it relates to how they see an individual, because your experience can be completely different. She would often see where I was scheduled and asked me how things were going. That short interaction would make my day. The saying is true: people will always remember how you made them feel. A few months went by and no fifth floor. Even though I felt bad for not going to see her, I would make excuses as to why it was okay for me not to. For example, I wanted to remember her as I knew her; my day was extremely busy; I had to stay on my unit; I had something to do after work—excuses, excuses, excuses. The bottom line was that I did not want to see her that way. I just could not imagine it.

One day when I agreed to work an off shift, I noticed my name was assigned to the fifth floor. There had to be a mistake. I informed the supervisor that I could not work that unit. My time had run out: I was either going to report to the unit or decide to quit at that moment. My supervisor explained to me that she kept me off the unit as long as she could. She went on to say that employees were complaining that they needed a break from the fifth floor, and of course they noticed that I had not rotated much. I wanted to be fair, as I stood there trying to decide. I immediately began to think that my supervisor granted a request that I made and now it was time for me to return the favor. I looked at my supervisor with my eyes watering trying to hold back tears and asked, "If I agree to go to the fifth floor, can I be assigned to the opposite side of the hall?" She said without any hesitation, "Of course." I felt better after she reassured me that I would not have to take care of my friend.

Even though she told me what I wanted to hear, when I went to the fifth floor, multiple emotions overtook me. I felt terrible because I was being selfish for not wanting to care for her. I was sad because being assigned to the fifth floor made me reminisce about the friendship we had. I was angry thinking about what happened to her. I felt ashamed because I was thankful and knew that it could have been me lying in that bed. It is amazing how we can easily take life, things and even people for granted. I never stopped to think how things must have been for her. What she felt like? What type of pain, discomfort or anguish she was experiencing? What she would be willing to give if she could have her life back? To be able to do everything she loved to do—dance, sing, play, laugh, run, jump, talk to her friends and family etc., etc., etc.

As the night went on everything in me wanted to go to her room. To my surprise, the unit was not as bad as I thought it would be. The assignment I had was very pleasant. The residents were quiet and very cooperative with the care that I provided for them. Some of them were bedridden while others were able to provide some assistance. I encountered no behavior issues and the team I worked with was amazing. There is nothing like working with individuals who understand that the overall goal was to take care of the patients first. I had a lot of down time and for every hour that went by I would try to walk to the other side of the unit to peek in on her, but each time I could not bring myself to do it. I was too nervous, and I could not go down that hallway despite my inner thoughts urging me to do so.

As my shift was coming to an end, I saw her mother. I wanted to keep walking as if I did not notice her getting off of the elevator, but I was too close. I knew she was going to want to talk, and within that conversation she was going to ask if I had seen her daughter. I was praying I would get called to do something or some type of emergency would arise. I was thinking this would be a great time for a fire drill, a call light, a phone call, or something. Instead, there was absolutely nothing. The unit was almost too perfect on this day. As she walked off the elevator, she recognized me, and I spoke. I asked her how she was doing, she asked me the same. As we proceeded to engage in small talk, she looked me directly in the eye and asked, "Have you had a chance to visit her yet?"

It was the question that I dreaded to hear. The "cat had my tongue" in that moment. My voice was stuck in my throat. I felt terrible and quickly ran a few crazy excuses in my head to give with the answer that I was about to say. I could barely look her in her eye with my head slightly bent I responded, "No I haven't." I tried to say that I had been very busy, but that sounded foolish and dumb seeing that I worked there. I had to face the fact that there were no excuses other than the fact that I was not ready and did not want to see her any differently than when she was healthy and full of life. I gave her my word that I would go see her, but I was not able to on that day. Deep down inside I could have seen her, but I was not sure what my reaction would be, and I did not want to have it with her mother in the room. As I was leaving the unit, I could hear her mother praying. She was a very spiritual woman, and I was told that she would come every day, sometimes with her grandson, and pray for hours at a time. I was determined to muster up the strength to go see her. I thought to myself that her mother was much closer to her than I was, and yet she gathered the strength to come see her daily while raising her grandson and dealing with the twists and turns that came with having an ill child suddenly. So I knew what my next move needed to be.

Life Lesson

Taking the time to be with someone
else in their time of need despite how
you feel can cause you to remember
that their lives have been impacted
in ways that you could not imagine.
You may have to sacrifice just an hour
or less when they have had to alter
life as they once knew it to be.

It's Bigger Than You

A week passed, and I was at the point that I was ready. I had heard a few things about her physical condition. I came face-to-face with my fears, and there was no looking back. One day I was asked to work over on the fifth floor, and I agreed. I was told that I was going to work the assignment that I was familiar with and could leave early if I would like to. I agreed to leave early, and I had made up my mind that I was going to use that time to go see her. Time went so fast it seemed unreal. It was 9:00 pm and I punched out, then went back to the floor and made my way to her room. She was not far from the nurses' station, but on the opposite side from where I was assigned. When I got off the elevator, I felt like I was walking in slow motion. As I approached her room, I took a deep breath and said to myself, "You can do this." As I walked in the room the covers appeared to be raised on her right side. As I drew closer, I noticed her right leg appeared bent toward her chest. My initial response was to turn back toward the door and cry. I had a moment and found myself sitting in a chair in her room and crying uncontrollably. I finally got it together somewhat, and stood beside her bed and told her repeatedly that I was so sorry. I was sorry for not coming to see her sooner. I was sorry for what had happened to her. I was sorry for making my feelings the priority and not being considerate as to what she must have gone through. I was just sorry for everything. The aide who was assigned to her walked into the room and asked if I was okay. I told her that I was and gave her the history between the patient and me. She gave me some reassurance and said, "You know now is better than never." That made me feel a little better. She went on to tell me that she came in to check her before her shift ended. She asked me if I could assist her. Of course, I agreed.

As she pulled the covers back, I was able to see her physical condition. Her left leg was contracted, stiff in a straight position with her foot plantar flexed (bent forward toward the bed) with the bone on the top of her foot protruding out with the skin intact. The right leg was also contracted. It was positioned toward her chest and the left side of her head was sunken in. She also had a tracheotomy, and I had to hold it together. She was the first trach patient that I had ever cared for or assisted someone with. I remembered how when we turned her, I initially jumped back because I did not realize how the sputum would protrude out of the trach when coughing. We had to get the nurse, because the coughing spell that she had, required that the nurse give her oxygen. Her coughing ceased and we proceeded to change her. She was cleaned, repositioned and made comfortable. I stayed after the assigned aide left the room. There on her table was a picture of the person I knew. I told her that I was going to come back and see her, and I did just that.

I got to the point that I looked forward to going to the fifth floor even when I was not assigned to it just to go in and check on her. I was told that she was in a vegetative state, but there were times that I questioned that. I had gotten to the point that when I would visit her, I would read or reminisce about the earlier years and tears would come from her eyes. To me it was a sign that she was still in there somewhere. I could not wait to see her mom and let her know that I had gone to see her. One day when I was in her room, her mother walked in. We smiled and shared a long-needed hug. I had the opportunity to meet her grandson for the first time. When I saw him looking at the bed and he called out, "Mama," I broke down again. Her mother said to her, "Girl, you have to get out of this bed. That boy is trying to take this baby from me." It was painful to hear and watch. I had to excuse myself from the room. I can honestly say that I had conquered my fears, and I made it a priority that every time I was scheduled to work, she would see my face. I kept my word, and the staff knew that if I were in the room and she needed anything I would take care of it. I began to truly understand the power of giving. I was given the opportunity to care for my friend in her time of need. The more time I spent with her, the more comfortable I became. I was so in tune with her that I knew when she was going to have a coughing episode or was in pain. The nurses were always like "Johnny on the spot" to make sure her needs were met. I became accustomed to working on any unit that I was rotated on. I understood that the quality of work was to remain the same regardless of where I was assigned.

It was a Thursday morning, and I will never forget this day for as long as I live. I was scheduled to work on the fifth floor. I was not assigned to care for my friend, but I did go to her room to speak to her and let her know that I was working the unit. There were two other aides assigned to the unit with me. We were down one aide due to a call-off. There came a time within the shift when the aides that I was working with had to leave the unit. I had to cover their assignments, which entailed answering call lights, assisting residents as needed, as well as the nurses with any specifics that were requested. I was not prepared for what was about to occur. The nurse reported that the patient in room 511 was transitioning. I thought to myself, *Did she say what I think she said?* Maybe she had the rooms mixed up. I had just been in the room and I did not notice anything. Then I thought maybe she had the wrong room number. My stomach was upside down and I felt numb. I counted to 100 and slowly made my way down the hall. I began to wonder if the other two aides were coming back. I wondered to myself what in the world was going on. What could have changed that fast? I had been in her room less than two hours before. My head was spinning uncontrollably. I was afraid, upset and nervous all at the same time. I would have preferred not to be there during that time. I was very nervous and did not want to accept what I was hearing. I slowly walked down the hall, looked in her room and noticed that she had oxygen on and was sweating. I walked in the room, cried, and could not allow myself to stay. I had never experienced a death as a healthcare provider. This was completely different. I was not ready for it. The one thing healthcare had taught me on this day was that, despite not being ready, the needs of others supersede yours. Neither of the aides had returned to the unit and the nurse informed me that assistance was needed. I recalled seeing the nurses and supervisor coming out of the room. They all looked sad and a few of them were crying. I heard one of them say that her mom would be there shortly. She had passed away and I had to assist the nurse in postmortem care. I took a deep breath and proceeded with tears in my eyes to clean her up and make her presentable for when her family arrived. Some of the staff members from the other units came in and assisted me.

I felt like things were moving in slow motion. I began to reminisce about our childhood years as I washed her face, then I glanced at the picture that sat on the nightstand. It was a picture of her in a blue dress with a huge, beautiful smile, her hair in curls, her hands folded on her lap as she sat in the famous wooden wicker chair. She did not have a care in the world. It was at that moment that I wished I had the power to change the hands of time. My thoughts were filled with could have, would have, and should have. If only I could have spent more time with her. If only I would have said, "I love you as a friend." If only I would have hugged her to let her know that I cared. All kind of thoughts were rushing through my head, including how hard this was for me. The experience could never be erased. When I finished cleaning her up, I held her hands for a while and told her that I was so sorry that her life had to end this way. As I released her hand and walked toward the door, I stopped in the doorway and said to myself, "God, if I can do this, I can do anything."

This was my moment of impact. I did not see this coming. Despite being tremendously hurt, I was determined to go to school and pursue a career in which I could dedicate my life to helping others.

Have you ever been hesitant to visit someone who has experienced a health challenge? If so, why?

____

____

____

____

What are some feelings that you have experienced when dealing with a loved one's illness and how did you cope with them?

____

____

____

____

Life Lesson

Never take the people in your life for granted. Remember that life is a gift, and it is not a promise. Let everything you do for someone else be on purpose.

What has been the most difficult situations that you have had to press through, and what were three key things that helped you through it?

____

____

____

____

Have you ever had a situation in your life that influenced you to do more than what you were doing at that time? If so, explain:

____

____

____

____

The Evolution of a Wounded Soul

It was time for a change, and I needed to see myself in a different place. I had to build myself up to tackle my fears, take control of my negative thoughts, and push toward a place that was foreign, by yelling out consistently, *"Why not you?"* That was a scary feeling, especially when there was not a strong push to do better and further my education.

There were several nurses that I would talk to, to inquire about nursing school, the expectations, the requirements, and the amount of time that it would take. I learned several things as I was gathering information:

1. Every experience is different.

2. You cannot share your desires, dreams, or goals with everyone.

3. You will gain haters along the way.

4. If it is something you really desire to do, you will take the time to make it happen.

I realize gossip can spread quickly. It was like being in high school all over again. There were several nurses and nurse aides that would talk to me just to confirm if I was considering going to school to become a nurse. It was crazy, because their primary motive was to discourage me from taking the steps to better myself. I heard multiple stories how either they or people they knew flunked out of nursing school, how difficult it was to get in, how the program itself was difficult and was designed to limit the percentage of blacks – as they put it – out of the program. I got to the point of not sharing much even when I was asked questions.

I learned how to have goals, dreams, and desires, and to limit my conversation with individuals that I knew had my best interest at heart. My circle was small but loyal. During this time, I was living with a very special soul that was powerful in her own way. She stood approximately 5'5", was very conservative, organized, and smart, and had a warm spirit. Annie Givens gave me some of the fundamental tools that equipped me to see beyond where I was. Her name changed from Ms. Givens to "Mom". We shared a lot and spent quality time with each other. She was the one who taught me how to balance a check book. She gave awesome advice, and the thing I can appreciate the most was that she always allowed me to make my own decisions. She was a great supporter, she was patient, she believed in me and she saw me as her daughter. She truly was my Shero! I can recall the day I sat down with her at the dining room table and shared my thoughts about going to school to become a nurse. I had decided to go to IVY Tech State College to become an LPN (Licensed Practical Nurse). It was a one-year program, from January 1992 to December 1992. I thought to myself, *How am I going to do this full-time?* As I was pondering, she stated, "You're not going to be able to work." It was as if she heard my thoughts. She then said, "You don't have to work if you are going to school." When I think about that moment in time, it brings tears to my eyes, because I know that it was nothing but God – that despite the situation I was in, he had someone in my life who was willing to take a chance on me. I could not explain it; all I knew was that I had to prove I was worth the investment, I was serious about my future and determined not to let anything, including the negative people, discourage me.

I registered at IVY Tech Gary Campus several months prior to the start date for the LPN program. I had to take several remedial courses because I did not score high enough on the entrance exam. To this day I think it was more because of my nerves than anything. After I got over that hurdle, it was time for me to take the entrance exam for the actual program. I studied and prepared as if my life depended on it. Regardless of where I was, I would read, and if I was not clear on something, I would read some more. The exam was something that I could not explain. The questions were so unrelatable that I could not determine if I passed it or not. I was numb and had made up my mind that if I did not pass, I would take it again. Somehow, some way, I passed! It was a very joyful day for me.

I had made up my mind that I was going to do this. I was the youngest in the class and I did not hesitate to get to know my classmates. I had a very strong support group. Cindy, Latrice and Debbie were the type of women that made sure everyone was okay, and if there was a need they did not mind helping. We looked out for each other, and it was amazing. We spent many nights, studying all night to make sure everyone comprehended the information. I often say that, out of all the schooling that I have had, IVY Tech was the toughest. The instructors were old school and made sure that you knew the information – they did not play. Mrs. Daneil wore high heels every day. She had a walk that was out of this world. You could hear her heels as she walked down the hall. We always knew when she was on the scene. She was incredibly knowledgeable. She would teach as if you already knew the information. I remember wondering how in the world I was going to keep up. I had to study with everything that was in me. Having her as an instructor was one of the reasons the study group existed. She was the type of instructor that if you asked a question, you would most likely end up doing a research paper on the question asked and would have to present it to the class. So, you caught on quickly to research before asking or write your question down and look up the information during your study time, because it was much easier. Ms. Love was genuine, very soft-spoken and could put you in your place without ever raising her voice. I admired that about her.

I recall lining up for clinicals. If you wore a dress, you had to literally get on your knees, and if your dress did not touch the floor you had to leave. If your nails were over your fingertips, you had to leave. If you were five minutes late you had to leave. If your uniform was not bleached white you had to leave. If your shoes or stockings were dirty you had to leave. If your underwear were not black you had to leave. We were to wear stud earrings only, hair up – *never* hanging – and it was a must that you wore the famous nurse hat. She made sure IVY Tech College of Gary Indiana was represented well. The word "excuse" was not in her vocabulary. Mrs. King had her approach with all the students, and made sure that when she taught, you listened. She wanted you to understand the information, not just learn it for the test. She had a way about herself that demanded attention. Mrs. King had two teeth missing in the front and had a short stature, but everyone knew not to take it for granted. She was a powerhouse in her own way.

Ms. Tuner taught pharmacology, and for some reason it was very difficult for me to grasp. Despite studying very hard,

I was not getting it. I was not sure if it was me or how it was being taught. Either way, I decided to make the decision to drop out and return the following semester because it was a challenge for me. Mrs. Horn was the program director. I spoke to her concerning the next semester classes. I asked if pharmacology was going to be offered and who was going to teach it. The way the program was designed was that if you did not pass specific classes you had to wait until it was offered again then proceed with the remainder of the classes. Pharmacology was one of those classes. I never spoke to Mrs. Horn about the decision that I made because my plan was to make sure my ducks were in a row, and I had a clear understanding of what I needed to do. As I was giving my plan strong consideration to give up, quit and to return to school later, I found out I was pregnant. This changed the entire trajectory of my life, my plans, my thoughts as well as my decision. To this day I look at it as the realm in the bush. This truly was my saving grace. It gave me the pick-up that I needed to push through the challenge and position myself to where I began to sleep, eat, talk, and live pharmacology. I remembered why I started this journey in the first place. I was determined that my life was not about just me, but the life that I was carrying deserved better. The study group that I had made sure no one was left behind. I saw myself passing. I had many days when I would look in the mirror and say to myself, "You can do this, do not stop, do not give up, just do not quit." It was rough, but I did it. I learned what it means to encourage yourself.

I had heard from some of the students that if you got pregnant, they would kick you out of the program. I never heard this from instructors, and I never told them. I hid my pregnancy very well. I carried small and I never had to wear maternity clothes. My Kourtney, despite her knowledge at that time, gave me the momentum, the strength, and the push that I so desperately needed at a time when I was ready to throw in the towel. My circle were the only ones that knew I was pregnant. Toward the end of my last few months, I began to show. I was nervous because I truly believed that they were going to kick me out of the program. Ms. Love pulled me to the side one day in clinical and asked me if I was pregnant. I looked at her, tearing up with my eyes full of fear, and answered, "Yes, I am." I just knew that was it. I had got so close, but now it was all going to end.

To my surprise, she said, "Well, if that is the case, we should break for lunch so you can get something to eat."

I had been worried for nothing!

During my pediatric rotation I had an instructor that was very judgmental and not as connected to the students as the other instructors. I was very well pregnant, and my belly was out there. She pulled me to the side to give me my evaluation. The evaluation was good, but she said something that I will never forget. She said, "You will never go beyond being an LPN." To this day I do not know why she made that comment. Was it because I was pregnant, because I was young, because I was African American, or because I was all three? Who knows? I did not question, dispute, or report what she said to me. It stung, but it did not stay! The other instructors were very supportive. I graduated pregnant and all, on December 10, 1992. I had my daughter December 26, 1992. Even though I was physically carrying my daughter, little did she know she was carrying me.

Life Lesson

When you think you are at your breaking point and ready to throw in the towel, reach down deep, pull from that undiscovered hidden place that only God can give, to help you press through that hopelessness to regain focus toward a goal that you can see.

Life Lesson

Never allow an individual to speak their version of your destiny to stop your growth. Instead, know what you are made of and press to move mountains to get to where you want to be.

Have you ever had to see yourself different from where you were? If so, explain:

____

____

____

____

What was it about an individual that helped motivate you to push toward something you were passionate about?

____

____

____

____

What have you done that required the support of others to get through it?

____

____

____

____

Have you ever had someone say something negative that was intended to limit your ability to move forward with your goals? If so, what was it and how did you handle it?

____

____

____

____

CHAPTER FIVE

The Road to Recovery

I gained a new view of myself when I graduated. I felt like I was given one of the most precious gifts ever: the ability to provide care and services to someone that was not able to care for themselves. I took the Florence Nightingale Pledge to heart as the candle I carried was lit. I stood up straight in my white uniform, stockings, shoes, and hat. The class consisted of approximately 17 students, and we all said the pledge in unison: "I solemnly pledge myself before God and in the presence of this assembly, to pass my life in purity and to practice my profession faithfully. I will abstain from whatever is deleterious and mischievous and will not take or knowingly administer any harmful drug. I will do all in my power to maintain and elevate the standard of my profession and will hold in confidence all personal matters committed to my keeping, and all family affairs coming to my knowledge in the practice of my calling. With loyalty will I endeavor to aid the physician in his work and devote myself to the welfare of those committed to my care. (Florence Nightingale Pledge, 1893)"

The one thing that resonated within me was that I had someone's life in my hands. That way of thinking never left me. I understood that my assignment was to gain as much knowledge as I could to be able to provide the best care possible and allow my patients to experience healthcare at its best. Several months after I had my daughter it was time for me to get a job. I worked as a graduate nurse as I prepared to take my state board to become licensed. My first nursing job was at East Chicago Rehab, which is a long-term care facility. It had two floors and consisted of skilled and intermediate residents. When they called me for the interview, I was extremely nervous. I could not sleep. I tossed and turned all night, thinking about the questions that I would be asked. This was my first job as a nurse, but I was more than ready to work! I wore a black skirt and jacket with a white shirt.

As I sat in the lobby my feet were tapping the floor, my heart was pounding, and I felt like I had a 20 lb. weight on my chest. It seemed like I had been waiting for hours but it was actually just a few minutes. Several residents would periodically come to the lobby area and asked me my name. Others would ask if I would be working there. I answered, "Well, we will see." Then I would tell them that I was there for an interview. I asked them how they liked living there. All the residents unanimously said that they liked it. That was a positive for me. Approximately 20 minutes passed, and I was told that the director was ready to see me. I stood up and walked to her office, which was several feet from where I was sitting. My legs felt like noodles. I did not know if it was from nerves or because I felt like I was waiting a long time, but I was not. I stood up and slowly walked to her office. In the first office that I passed, there was a woman in a suit who was upset about something. She was on the phone speaking very loudly. I quickly glanced in the room and on the outside of the door it read "Administrator's Office." When I walked past, she closed the door.

As I approached the second office the door read "Director of Nursing." She was dark complexioned, approximately 5'6", wore glasses and had a short blunt haircut that was tapered around her ears. Her name was Mrs. Moody. Even though I was nervous and had very little sleep I was ready to conquer this milestone in my life so I could begin my next journey. She asked me a few basic questions. I only had my high school experience as a certified assistant and nurse training to draw from. I did not have any nursing experience, but she seemed to like the answers that I gave. As I was interviewing, she asked me if I had just had a baby. I answered yes and asked her how she knew. She smiled and pointed at my shirt. I was extremely embarrassed. The front of my shirt was completely wet with breast milk. I had been so nervous about the interview that I forgot to put on the breast pads. I excused myself and went to the bathroom to clean up as much as possible and came back to complete the interview. She asked when I could start.

I was excited and ready to work. I noticed that working in the field did not always match how things were explained in the textbooks. Not every scenario was perfect like the book portrayed, and sometimes things had to be substituted for others. One day I had to give a resident an injection. I went into the room, introduced myself, and explained to the resident what I was going to do. I checked the resident's armband and verified that I had the correct person. I went to the cart and prepared the medication. When the mediation was prepared to be given, I went into the room and told the resident that I was back to administer his injection. As I aimed the needle at the resident's arm and was about to administer the medication, the fire alarm went off. He jumped up, swinging his arms and causing me to stick myself, while yelling, "What the hell is going on?" He demanded that I get out of his room. It was like I was co-starring in a scene of *Grey's Anatomy*. I was trying to process everything. I did not recall reading about this in the textbook. That was the very moment that I discovered that your day can be very unpredictable. I may have had things planned out in my head one way, but it was clear that situations can arise that are totally out of your control. Later I found out that he served in the war and would have outbursts and aggressive episodes whenever he heard loud noises. I thought to myself, *Is that not something you would want to inform someone of, especially a new nurse?* "Hey people help me out here!" I felt more than eaten at that moment, I felt devoured. I was told in report that there was nothing new with him and he was okay. Everything turned out well with me. I was not physically hurt, just emotionally bruised a bit and a little upset. I remembered asking the three million-dollar why questions: Why was I not told about his behavior? Why was his room located so close to the alarms? Why was the drill not announced, especially after finding out that they were just testing the system? I was truly taken off guard. I was not advanced enough to have thought to even look at the care plan or ask about care cards. I quickly learned the importance of knowing your residents as well as giving and receiving a thorough report. My director would always check on me just to make sure I was okay. She would see me with a resident and say to me, while patting me on my back, "You are doing a good job." She was very encouraging, positive and would let me know that her door was always open.

I found myself having to do certain things that I had not experienced as a student. Most of the nurses were very patient with me, but there were a few nurses that really did not want to be bothered with training a new grad. I can recall thinking, *everybody had to have a starting point regardless of what type of job they have.* There is a saying that nurses "eat their young," and in some cases it is true. It's never a good feeling to be in a new place, with no experience, and needing to be trained, developed and mentored, and what you get in return is attitude, someone who is working at their pace to get things done because they want to leave on time, or those who complain to their co-worker that they don't have time to train. When there were things that I was not familiar with and wanted to make sure certain procedures were done appropriately, I would ask for assistance.

One day as I was walking toward the front lobby area, the business office manager and another office employee heard about me asking for help. They pulled me to the side and said, "You need to stop saying that you don't know and asking people to explain things to you." My first thought was, *I know they did not interrupt my day with this foolishness*, and I counted to ten before I responded. I was very respectful and professional. I was 23 years old, and they were in their mid- to late-50s. I had to take a deep breath and explain to them my views as they related to my career. I recall explaining that I understood the seriousness of my job: I had someone's life in my hands, and one mistake could cost them their life. I made it clear that I would rather be safe than sorry. I was more concerned about my resident's outcome than my pride. It's sad to say that the two individuals who did not have a clue of the responsibility that I had felt that they had a right to say what I should stop doing because of how it looked. I had to walk away and realize people have the right to their opinion, but I have the final say, and therefore of whether I was going to allow their opinion to affect me. That conversation went in one ear and out of the other. I refused to give it any energy.

I was learning a lot and was very careful not to make mistakes. My director would periodically give me what I would call "professional nuggets". She would say things like, "Always make rounds and get to know your residents. Never rely on everything that is said and take time to do your own assessment. Always respond to a concern that the aides report because they will in many cases notice a change in a resident's condition first." She would have me stop by her office and share her nursing experiences with me. It was as if she took me under her wing and made me her focus project. Several months had passed and she asked me to meet her in her office. I immediately thought she wanted to have one of her encouraging or meaningful nursing talks, but that was not the case. This time when she asked me to come to her office it was different. She did not seem as relaxed as she normally was. It was the end of the day and conversations normally took place during the shift. I started to think to myself, *I hope everything is ok*. I had taken everything to heart that had ever been spoken to me. I knew all the residents by name. I would make rounds so I could visually put my eye on every resident for whom I was responsible. I would ask multiple questions if more information were needed so I could get a clear understanding of what was going on with the patients. I took pride in my role and wanted my work to exemplify that. As I sat in her office, she began to compliment me on what she had been hearing and what she observed. I was tapping my feet wondering, *Okay where is this going? Is she going to fire me because I do not have my license? Has the graduate nurse working program been canceled and she is trying to let me down easy?* I was worried and said to myself, "Can we please just get to the point: if you have to let me go just say it." I honestly did not know what to think.

My first response was to think negatively. I knew that I needed money because I had another mouth to feed. While I was in nursing school, I was receiving government assistance. I wanted to be able to carry my own weight to some degree. Ms. Givens (Ma) provided a roof over my head and paid all the bills. I felt the least I could do was to pay for the groceries. I did not want to depend on the system. I wanted to make my own way. I had planned to get the assistance that I was eligible for, finish school, get a job, then come off. I remembered once having to break a penny bank open and look between couches for loose change to get money for milk because my WIC was delayed. I was determined to make a good life for myself and not allow my children to have to experience any of the financial hardships that I had. As I was sitting in the office, she spoke for over 15 minutes, then she reached on the side of her computer and got some papers. I just knew they were termination papers. My heart was beating fast, and I started to tear up a bit. She placed the papers in front of me, and the top page had black bold typing on it. It read "Restorative nurse program." To my surprise, it was the opposite of what I thought she wanted to say to me. She went on to explain that there was a new program called restorative nursing, and she wanted me to develop it. I was initially shocked, hesitant, and speechless, because there were nurses who were way more qualified than I was, and they had a license. I thought this was crazy! What did she see in me that I did not see in myself? I felt that I was too new to develop anything. I was still trying to make sure that I was being developed. I did not even have a license! She must have been thinking about someone else, because I felt that I was not the one. I had no idea what this program entailed. I expressed to her that I had a lot to learn and that I was not ready to be responsible for a program of any kind. She asked me to at least think about it, and gave me her word that if I would reconsider, she would make sure I had everything I needed and would be 100% supportive. She then gave me the information she had and asked me to review it. She never pressured me or asked me about the position again. She was serious when she said she was going to let me take my time, review the information, and think about it. Several weeks passed, and I reviewed what the program entailed. Then, despite my fears, hesitancies and uncertainty, I expressed to her that I would take the position.

Having the clarity of knowing that someone's life is in your hands should allow you to move your pride to the side. Choose to humble yourself to gain wisdom and understanding in areas that you have no knowledge. The saying is true: sometimes you don't know what you don't know.

Life Lesson

Remember, we all had to start somewhere. Training is an essential part of development in any field. Never forget where you started and who helped you along the way. "Eating our young" is a sad statement, but true. People often forget that they were once the young, but dismissed the fact that they made it because someone else gave them the time and attention to become who they are today.

Have you ever taken a pledge or committed to something and settled within yourself that you were going to see it through? If yes, explain what it was, and if not, explain why it was not completed.

____

____

____

____

If you have ever interviewed for a position, what were some key things you recalled that either helped you get the position or the reason you believe you were not chosen.

____

____

____

____

How have you stopped other individuals' opinions from distracting you from obtaining goals or knowledge despite what was said?

Explain what training you have had and evaluate a person who trained you. If they had the opportunity to train you again, would you welcome it? Why or why not?

Have you ever taken a position that you did not feel qualified for? If yes, what was the position, explain why you agreed to take it, and what was the outcome?

Walk By Faith

Despite what I was feeling internally I took on the challenge to develop this program that I know very little about. I had a conversation with my director and explained to her what I understood from the information that she provided me. I explained to her that from my understanding I had to develop a team that would focus on keeping the residents as functional as possible via AROM (active range of motion) – meaning the resident was capable of moving their own extremities – or PROM (passive range of motion) – meaning the resident required someone to move their extremities for them. It would involve eating programs, identifying residents who had contracture (stiffness with difficulty to no extension of their extremities), assessments. and of course, documentation. These were just a few of the processes required. There was an entirely different section that I had not explored. I was not certain how this assignment was going to work out for me. I did not have anyone who I could bounce things off of to verify that the program was being developed correctly, because everyone was trying to grasp the new concepts and processes related to the requirements. What I did understand clearly was that I needed a starting point. I gathered binders and organized the residents in groups based on the assessments that were done. My director did have a licensed nurse assigned to do the assessments. That was a relief for me, because what continued to rush through my head was that I did not have a license.

I formulated an interview questionnaire to recruit the aides that were to assist me. It focused on their work ethics, professionalism, attendance, their ability to get along with others, personality and documentation abilities. Prior to me implementing any process I always got the approval from the director to verify if there was anything she wanted to add or give further guidance and assurance that I was doing things correctly. I was clear that I was in a very fragile developmental stage, and the experience I gained from this employer could either enhance my professional outlook on my career or it could put a black mark of disappointment that could leave unwanted scars.

I had spoken to many nurses on my journey, and discovered that some nurses are in the profession, but the profession is not in them. What I observed was that they had allowed experiences that they have had throughout their career to detour the passion they once had for the profession. In most cases when people think of nurses, they normally think of words like "compassionate", "caring", "considerate", "sacrifice" and "empathetic", to name just a few. The tragedy is that, once one has loss one's passion and has forgotten the true essence of what one's profession means and stands for, the opportunity presents itself to allow black marks to hinder the growth and development of those who are trying to navigate and find themselves in the maze of their new-found career.

Regardless of the experiences that awaited me, the one thing that stayed on the forefront of my mind was that my patients came first. I did get the approval for the interview form and I proceeded to interview. It was important to me that my director and I were on the same page with decisions that were being made. This was a highlight for me, because I had never interviewed anyone in my life for a job. The experience was rewarding. I had my small corner office cleaned and well organized. My uniform was fresh, clean, and ironed with a crease in my pants that did not move when I walked. I think I was more nervous than I needed to be. Once I started speaking to the candidates, my nerves eased and I allowed myself to lighten up a bit. I believed it was because I had worked with them within the facility, and they took the opportunity as well as the interview just as serious as I did. I selected two individuals that were perfect for the role.

A lesson that I learned early on was that some individuals have what I would describe as entitlement issues. There was one person who was the opposite of what I was looking for. She was always late, had to be constantly reminded to document, was argumentative with other staff members and had a few write-ups. I was initially shocked to see her name listed to be interviewed. I could not turn her away because the position was posted, and everyone was given the opportunity to be interviewed if desired. I later discovered that this individual was related to the nurse who was assisting me. OMG! What an awkward position I was in. A plan had been made, but I was excluded. The plan was for the employee to be transferred to the restorative department so she could work closer with her family member who would have been able to cover and attempt to protect her from getting into further trouble. The director had warned me about this individual. The employee was discussed prior to the interview and it was predetermined that she did not qualify for the position. Despite the uncomfortableness of the situation, I was clear that in order for the department to move in the right direction, the requirements had to be met and individuals that were selected had to be ready, willing, and able to work professionally and independently. Of course, the nurse who was assisting me had an issue with several things: she was doing the assessments, she had the license, she had been there longer, she was older and according to her I should have hired who she wanted in the department. I agreed with all these points, excluding the last issue mentioned. I never expressed to her that the director and I had a conversation concerning the unprofessional behavior of which she was already aware. In my opinion that was not for me to share. I was willing to take the heat and not hide behind a conversation. This gave me the opportunity to open up and express myself with the hopes that she would see the importance of what we were attempting to accomplish as a team. Instead, I explained to her our goals, and the reliable and professional staff we needed to make the new program work. She agreed with hesitancy.

I didn't realize it in that moment, but I had begun to establish within myself the importance of not being moved or influenced by things others may have felt needed to be done based on their personal motives. I had initially questioned why I was interviewing and asked to take on such a role instead of the nurse who was assisting me. As time went on it became clear. I learned very quickly several key factors that would never work to produce growth and teamwork. She had the type of character that she believed saying what she thought and felt was the best approach with everything. It was not that the message was sometimes needed, but the tone in most cases was demeaning, rude and inappropriate. It was obvious who were her favorites. The aides and nurses that she liked were treated very differently from the ones she did not. They were treated very professionally with smiles, nice gestures, and all positive vibes. Regardless of what they did – from coming in late, forgetting to document, inappropriate behavior or whatever else – they were always given a pass without a reprimand or barely a spoken word.

Charles Jones, the pastor I quoted earlier, would often say, "More is caught than taught." This was truly the case for me. I learned key principles that would reduce the morale, effectiveness, and growth of any establishment. One is that favoritism never works. It causes dissensions, separations, jealousies and overall a negative environment. Secondly, that giving guidance, instructions, reprimands or even corrections does not have to be done in a disrespectful way that is belittling and could cause offense. Several attempts had been made by the director to correct her behaviors, but from what I observed they were unsuccessful. I later understood why I was approached concerning the position: I was "moldable", as my director would put it. Initially, I did not know what she meant by that, but after she went on to explain I got it. I was very eager, excited, ready to learn, humble, open, fearful but ready to gain knowledge. I thought I was not ready for a leadership position, but despite me being new to nursing as well as this program it progressed. What I had come to realize was that regardless of what I was asked to do or where I was needed, I made myself available.

Working at this facility was very rewarding. I assisted in many different areas and was always willing to help. As time went on, I desired more. The nurses would often talk to me about finding my niche. The world of healthcare was so huge, and I wanted to discover just where I fitted in. I had to kick myself, because I was so busy working that I took for granted the time I needed to study for my exam. When I took it and did not pass, I was devastated and had no one but myself to blame. I had to buckle down and get my priorities together and pass the test that I needed to move forward, and I did just that. Approximately a year after I passed my boards I spoke to the director and the administrator together to inform them that I was seeking to go to the hospital. By this time, I had a new director of nursing – the previous director had become ill and was no longer able to work. They asked what they could do to get me to stay, but understood my reasons as to why I was going to leave. I was very appreciative of their understanding despite the pressure I felt to stay.

Change can be a positive thing, if it is embraced that a season has come to an end. I had reached that place within myself. Separation or detachment can be scary and many times it takes longer to do than desired because of the fear of the unknown or familiarity with a particular situation or career. A change of anything takes a new mindset, determination, time, energy, and outlook. It is not always easy, but it is obtainable. I know I had to make up in my mind to let go and explore or stay and remain stagnant. Separation or detachment is normally experienced before the physical act ever takes place. I experienced that professionally when the urge was within me to explore. I was not trying to build my resume, my name, or my reputation. I was much too new to even think on those things. I was trying to determine what avenue I needed to take to make a better version of myself. It was time to take a leap of faith. I had learned a lot of key things and felt that I had a good foundation. I had decided from the experience that I would never take on a key role while trying to reach a goal. At that time, the goal for me was obtaining my nursing license and developing as a nurse. I walked away with the door open just in case I wanted to return. I was taught years earlier by my store manager Mr. Larry, when I worked at the neighborhood grocery store, Valu Mart that you *never* leave a job the wrong way – always leave the door open just in case you ever need to return. He would end his statement by saying you never know what life is going to bring, and sometimes the people you meet going up are the same people you meet going down. What a powerful and true statement indeed! It is a life nugget that I live by to this day. I had an inner peace and at the same time excitement over the fact that my road to recovery was allowing me to not just gain insight about the profession, but about myself too.

I landed a job at Mercy Hospital in Gary, Indiana on the rehabilitation unit. Tencree Crawford was the director of nurses. There is something about having the faith and desire to learn and grow: God has a way of putting the right people in your path to motivate, push and encourage you to obtain what you have sought out to do despite the hiccups and disappointment that are experienced along the way. Tencree was amazingly knowledgeable and seemed to know everything as it related to fractures, wrappings, wound care, surgical procedure, care, etc. Her personality was stern and at the same time soft enough to where she was approachable and always willing to teach. She was open and would share her experiences with the hopes that the bigger picture was seen. The bigger picture was to always stay professional, the patients come first, follow up and ask questions to gain clarity when needed. The team was comprised of old school nurses, but not necessarily old.

Let me explain. The team of nurses were amazing. After report was given of the events from the previous shift, making rounds were automatic. Each nurse would check on their patients, introduce themselves and let them know to call if they needed anything. Rose was one of the nurses on the unit. She took pride in her patient care and wanted to always make sure everything was done. One day she had to leave work for an appointment. Within approximately 20 minutes of leaving, she called and made me aware that she had obtained an order for one of her patients to receive an IV. She sounded concerned but wanted to make sure the message was received so the patient could get his medication. The order was carried out and the patient IV medication was initiated. The next day, prior to getting a report, she went in to see the patient to ask how he was doing and was he feeling better. Her ultimate concern was that there was effective follow-through as well as the patient receiving proper care. Rose and I had met prior to working together and we studied together to pass our boards. What I respected the most is that she was always willing to listen to her patients and do everything she could to meet their needs. The true essence of a nurse! The nurses on the unit were bonded and always willing to assist each other. It was a wonderful thing to be a part of. The doctors were always friendly and took the time to teach and explain things as if you were their students. There were some nurses who wore the white traditional uniform, the nursing hat, stockings, white shoes, and all. They not only looked the part, they were the profession that they represented. Working with them really made me proud to have become a nurse even the more. My director would make frequent rounds on the unit to speak with the patient, evaluate their progression and to determine how they were doing overall.

One day as she was making rounds, she asked me to join her. As we proceeded to go into a patient's room that had recently had a bilateral amputation (the removal of both limbs either above or below the knee) she looked at me and said,

"I'm going to teach you everything I know." In that instant, I thought negatively and posed a question to myself: "Why me?" I had not been there long, she did not know me, what was the catch? I think about how quick I was to count myself out. I believe that it is a sense of security or lack thereof, when the initial take-away from something that is meant to be positive is automatically a negative thought. I had to ask myself why the initial take-away from her comment was not, "Why not me? I am worth the investment, I can be open to learn more, I can handle this." I know it was because I was still trying to find myself, my niche in the world of nursing. I was always open to learn, and the first to volunteer and demonstrate what was being taught to gain as much knowledge as I could. I was eager to explore but craved to be successful at it. My manager was true to her word, she did just as she said she would. She proceeded to explain and show me proper techniques relating to wrapping limbs on that same day. She removed the wraps of the patient who had just lost both limbs above the knee and had a bilateral amputation. She removed the wrap, one at a time. She began to explain the importance of circulation, how it is to be checked when a bandage is applied, the importance of proper documentation and always having the assurance that the wraps are done correctly. As she was completing wrapping the left stump, she says in a soft but stern voice, "Now I'm going to watch you do the other one." I was nervous but at the same time confident that I could do it. It was not the first time I had wrapped a stump. As she watched me very closely, she remained silent and assisted me by holding his stump so I could get underneath him to properly position the bandage and make sure the material was not folding. After the task was completed, she complemented me and said, "Nice job."

She reviewed my documentation and informed me that whenever she had anything that she wanted me to be exposed to, to enhance my knowledge or experience, she was going to make sure I was with her. She made sure I was clear on processes, techniques, and protocols. She literally took me with her and gave me experiences of a lifetime. Despite the fact that I was an LPN, and my role would limit me to performing specific duties, she made sure I had the exposure and was clear on how procedures were to be done. She showed me how to start an IV, administer a blood transfusion, mixing medications, flush PICC (peripherally inserted central catheter) lines and port-a-caths, etc. There was nothing that she was not willing to teach me. If it involved nursing and she was knowledgeable of it, she had no problem sharing the wealth. She was not only a director, but she was also a teacher and cared about if you understood the information given. She had patience to make sure you were clear and could explain things if ever needed.

There came a time when the hospital faced a challenging time with staffing. I was informed that the hospital had contracted several nurses from out of the country. The unit acquired several new nurses who were registered nurses (RNs) from the Philippines. She had me do some of the training.

One day as I was explaining a few procedures related to IVs and some of the machines that we used, she asked me to see her after I was done. I was not sure what she wanted. I initially thought that maybe she wanted to give me a few pointers on how to better explain things or a critique on how I left something out that needed to be clearer. I was pondering over what I might have done that she was requesting to speak to me, but I was not as nervous as before, because I had gained a trust and knew that she had my best interest at heart. I also knew that regardless of how she treated me, she had no problems correcting, confronting, or critiquing any matter if she felt it was needed.

I saw her walking in the hallway close by the room I was in with the nurses. I stepped out and asked if now was a good time. She said that it was, and I informed the nurses that I would be back. She did not take me out of view from where I was not able to see the nurses that I was training. She asked me to look in the room and tell her what I saw. In my head I said to myself, "Is this a trick question? What in the world is the point to this? This question has nothing to do with nursing." But I thought, *Okay,* and repeated the question to her: "What do I see in the room?"

She answered, "Yes, what do you see?"

I said, "I see two beds, the floor, an IV pole, three nurses, supplies, sheets, and curtains. Do you want me to keep going?"

"No, but go back to the three nurses."

"Okay?"

"What are they?"

"Females."

She smiled. "Profession – as it relates to their career. What are they?"

"Registered nurses."

"Who is training them?"

"I am."

"What is your title?"

"A licensed practical nurse."

Until that point, she had never separated the professional titles of an RN from the LPN. She looked me in the eye and said, "There is nothing wrong with you being an LPN, but there is more in you. I got you to train them for a reason. I wanted you to pull back for a moment to see your capabilities, to see how much you have grown, and to understand that the only thing that is separating them from you is a piece of paper." She had intense passion in her voice, and she made me feel that she wanted me to truly get what she was saying. She grabbed my arm as she continued to look me in the eye and said, "Baby girl, go back to school."

Some moments you will never forget, and for me this was one of those moments. I would talk about going back to school, but it was not a priority because I had become content. Despite having a desire, I was not focused enough to take action. That day changed everything: it pushed things into gear and gave me another prospective. It was what I considered to be the wakeup call I needed.

Life Lesson

Favoritism and demeaning behavior are
not characteristic of professionalism. They
are often a reflection of the disregard or
lack of awareness an individual has toward
how they are viewed by others.

Life Lesson

Being on the same page is important to prevent confusion, misunderstandings, and offenses. A clear understanding among all involved of the plan, the execution, and the goal is the key to better buy-in and a better outcome.

Life Lesson

Deciding to take on a new role should never only be about the money. What should matter is the dedication and level of commitment that one can give, with the goal being to make effective changes.

Life Lesson

Sometime the push you need is waiting
so it can be exposed from another
person or source to allow you to make
moves that you talked about but have
made no effort to truly act upon. Take
heed, take note, recognize, accept,
and take action. Why not you?!

Life Lesson

Never take for granted people who want to assist in your development. When experience wants to take you under their wings to give you more insight, knowledge and wisdom, know that it is a privilege and not an entitlement.

Have you ever witnessed behavior from a person in authority that was unfair or demeaning to a subordinate? If yes, what was it and how did it make you feel?

____

____

____

____

Give three characteristics that you feel should be displayed by a leader.

____

____

____

____

What have been some reasons you have decided to seek other employment, and how did you leave?

____

____

____

____

What do you feel may be reasons why people decide to continue to stay where they are despite the push or the desire they may have to do better?

____

____

____

____

If you are someone who procrastinates or struggles as to what path you want to take, what do you feel like you need at this point to get you moving in the direction that you desire to be in?

____

____

____

____

CHAPTER SIX

You Are the Expert of Your Own Life

Several months passed and I took the needed steps to stop talking about it and start being about it. The words and the intentional visual she allowed me to see through my own eyes were powerful, enlightening and so strategically done. To think I had no idea of the magnitude of information that I was sharing, to the point that it never dawned on me what was being observed by her and the potential that she saw in me. The way I saw it was that I was just doing what was asked. Little did I know that she was setting me up in a good way to really allow me to see me as more valuable than I had. It caused me to question myself and ask why I had not been back to school. Was I stuck in a place of comfort? Had talking about a goal become satisfying because it seemed like the right thing to say? What was keeping me from moving forward? Was I afraid to fail? Was I a procrastinator who had become complacent where I was, or did I not feel like putting in the time?

I had to have a moment with myself to analyze where I was mentally, what I was going to do, and determine what was needed to get there. In that moment I made up my mind that I was going to take action, make moves and make things happen. I had spoken about attending Indiana University Northwest (IUN) prior to enrolling. I had come to the realization that no one could do it for me, so I had to have a ready set mind to make a committed decision to become the change agent in my own life. I decided to enroll at Indiana University Northwest campus. When I attended IVY Tech, I would say that I knew one day I would like to continue my education and would attend Indiana University for my RN. That day had finally come! Despite the fact that I had to be reminded by a strategy that I never saw coming, the plan worked. When I enrolled in school it took me back to my IVY Tech days, trying to finish one program and talking about another. I thought to myself, "Boy, time flies." I was excited about finally doing what I was at one time only talking about. It was a great feeling to be acting upon a thought, a conversation and a vision that was finally coming to fruition.

Before I enrolled, I spoke with my family to explain to them the level of commitment, dedication and sacrifice that was going to be needed, in order to complete the program. I had married shortly after my LPN program, and during that time it was important that any decisions made were agreed upon. The stamp of approval was given, and it was time for the true test to begin.

Day one was intense but there was no looking back. The instructor, who stood about 6'2", was slim and with short hair, started his class by saying how we had made a choice of a lifetime and things would not be easy. He went on to say that all requirements needed to be met to move on to the next phase of whatever program we had selected. I said to myself, "Dang, we just walked into the door!" My seat had not even warmed up from me sitting in it. I was thinking, *Okay, this is serious business!* Of course, I knew before I got there that it was, I just had never had anyone who was very direct and matter of fact, with a no apparent personality or interest in consoling the scared and uncertain faces of some of the individuals that were in the class. It was not until I heard his introduction that I became nervous. I began to look around at the room and I noticed that it was full of individuals of all ages. There were older individuals that were returning students, those that were fresh out of high school and of course the young adults. Everyone seemed to be excited, nervous, and ready to see what was expected in the days ahead. The initial classes that I had to take were required college courses. My instructors were very straightforward, and the expectations of the classes were spelled out via the syllabus. I was doing well, taking the time needed to study and passing all the required courses. I was making it happen, working my way down the finish line to get to the end of the initial requirements.

Toward the end of the semester there was a shift. My body, or should I say my stomach started to react very strangely to certain foods that I once enjoyed eating. When I would go to the cafeteria or walk past someone eating, I would feel a case of slight nausea, but it would subside when I got out of the vicinity of the smell. The first time the nausea occurred I did not think anything of it, but the more I noticed it the more concerned I became. I was still working at the hospital and things were going great. I was working, going to school with a goal in mind and a plan to get there. I would speak to a few of my co-workers about the symptoms I was having, and they would jokingly ask, "Are you pregnant?" My response was always the same "Pregnant, absolutely not!" In all honesty being pregnant had crossed my mind, but refusing to truly consider it allowed me to ignore that possibility. If that was not a crazy way of thinking at that time! Now think about it: me being a nurse should have ruled out that possibility immediately. It did not excuse the fact that I would have days when I did not feel my best, so being the nurse that I was I had to begin the assessment phase to rule out what the heck was going on. I remember being at my apartment with a test in my hand taking multiple rapid deep breaths and saying to myself, "Maybe it is an ulcer, maybe I need to use the restroom, maybe I was eating food that was disagreeing with my stomach." I went on and on trying to think of every excuse in the book. It seemed like the hallway from the front door to the restroom was thousands of feet long. It was like the room had stopped and I was moving in slow motion. That moment felt like the Spike Lee movies when he would have the special effects and the person would be moving up toward the screen, but they were not actually walking. It was as if they were gliding on a slow, moving conveyor belt as they were in a standing position. Despite the fact that the bathroom was only approximately six steps away, it felt like a very long journey. I took the test and it showed exactly what was being said. All I knew was on that day I met the world record of taking the longest shower in the world. I had a few weeks before the end of the semester. I completed two semesters and decided to drop out until after the baby was born.

To this day I cannot explain my action. I was able to tolerate being nauseated every now and then. I did not have any other symptoms, apart from occasional tiredness. I was still working at the hospital, so to this day I cannot explain or rationalize what made me decide to stop going to school. In my head now I say, "Deb, you were only just pregnant." It's strange how life can be moving in one direction, and things change. It is in those crucial moments when the unexpected occurs that seeking out wise counsel or not being quick to make decisions can be crucial to one's future, finances, or other important aspects in life that need to be clearly thought out, planned, and taken into consideration. I had made a decision that did not make rational sense, but for some reason it was made. I had made a vow to myself that I was going to return to school no matter what. I continued working, and the moment had come when I needed to have the uncomfortable conversation with my manager. I had concluded in my own head that the conversation was going to be negative, because of the disappointment that I thought she was going to have toward me. As I walked into her office and sat down, I said, "You are not going to like what I am about to say." A tear rolled down my face and she asked with such overwhelming compassion, "What's wrong?" I began to explain that I was pregnant and decided to put school on hold until after the baby was born. She looked into my eyes and said, "You will be fine, I know you will." She grabbed my hand and gave it a gentle squeeze. It was comforting and reassuring at the same time. The brief but needed conversation was the total opposite of what I had imagined it would be. I was stressing over a few words that took less than 20 minutes. There was no judgment, she never made me feel uncomfortable, embarrassed, or stupid for making the decision that I did. I appreciated the fact that she allowed my decision to be my decision, regardless if she felt, believed, or thought differently. Her response was so authentic that her thinking any differently never crossed my mind. Her response made me feel even stronger about not just letting her down but, more importantly, letting myself or my unborn child down.

I continued to grow and sharpen my skills. Mercy Hospital had a family-like environment. The doctors would visit the units and at times bring food. When the unit came together to have lunch, it was always very enjoyable and welcoming. The staff was very professional and friendly. It was a good environment to work in and the morale was very positive. Being a nurse and working in the same hospital as my obstetrician had its perks, but it also had its downfalls. My obstetrician would make rounds periodically and would always greet me with a huge smile and ask, "How are you doing?" He would remind me often not to overdo it. My response was always the same, "Doc I'm doing fine, all is well!"

Several months had passed, and I was coming down to the wire. As time went on, I noticed I was getting bigger by the day, which is a normal response to pregnancy. I was more belly than anything. I had no issues working, and I was not having any discomfort, apart from a slight swelling of my feet from being on them all day. Other than that, I was able to go about my daily duties with no issues. My prenatal visits were going great. I was getting tired and looking forward to not being pregnant. I would always get reminders to take it easy, not overdo it, get my rest, and make sure I was eating. It was clear that I had no issues in that department.

One day I was taking care of an elderly gentlemen that had multiple medical issues. By this time, I was a few weeks from my delivery date. I went into the room and introduced myself and explained to him that I was going to be his nurse for the day. I reviewed his case after getting report from the previous nurse, who stated that he had an uneventful night. In other words, he had no concerns or issues with his care and overall, he had a comfortable and restful night. He was alert and oriented to person, place, time, and situation. His diagnosis included but was not limited to heart disease, diabetes, CVA, hypertension and a recent hip replacement secondary to a fall that he experienced at home. He was due to be discharged the next day. He was very pleasant and required minimal assistance. He had finished his physical therapy and his weight bearing was up as tolerated, his surgical site was healing very well, and he barely complained of any pain. He expressed to me that he was ready to go home to be with his wife. She had been ill but had fully recovered. He mentioned that when she came home from the hospital, he had his accident a few weeks later. He went on to say that not a day had passed on which he had not spoken to her. He would light up every time he said anything about her. It was the cutest thing to see how the mentioning of her made his day. He said that they had been married for over 40 years. I told him that was precious, and asked what was the secret to their longevity. He responded, "Well young lady, my wife has always let me run everything." I looked him in his eyes and said to myself, "Did he just say that?" He stopped me before I could think anything further and said, "I run the vacuum, bath water, errands – you name it, I make sure it is done." We laughed and laughed. He asked me how far along I was, and I told him in my ready to deliver voice, "I'm due in a few more weeks." He congratulated me and mentioned how he could not wait to see his grandchildren. I left the room and told him that I would be back with his medication.

Approximately 20 minutes passed, and he had his call light on. I went into his room and he stated that he needed to use the restroom. He had a bedside commode. As I went to move his leg, he said, "Maybe you should get someone else to assist you." I had been told in report of his physical abilities that he required minimal assistance. I did not think anything of it. I never thought it would pose a threat or concern to my physical condition. He stood up and placed his hand in mine for support as he slightly pivoted onto the seat. He called me back into the room and as he stood up, I noticed his balance was off. I reached him just in time before he slumped over onto the bed. I immediately placed his legs onto the bed and called a code blue. As my co-workers entered the room, they observed me initiating CPR. My obstetrician was making rounds at that time, and who did he see sweating and do-ing chest compressions before someone else took over? Yes, it was me. He immediately had me removed from the scene, checked out to make sure I was ok, and informed my direc-tor that I was starting my leave at that moment. Everything happened so fast. One minute I was talking to my patient who was doing well, anticipating going home to see his wife and grandchildren, and just like that he was gone. That expe-rience taught me that time is a precious commodity and to never take it for granted. This was my first time experiencing a condition change that rapidly, and death was the result. Can you imagine what was going through my mind? It was very upsetting! I had just had an extensive conversation with this individual who shared his expectations and plans but never had the opportunity to experience what he spoke about.

I was very professional yet compassionate. I followed the instructions that were given by my doctor. Before I left the hospital, I went back into my patient's room as the aides were preparing his body and I said a silent prayer for his family. That day I left the hospital in a mood that I could not explain. I had an experience that was life-changing and was preparing to have another experience of a lifetime. Several weeks had passed. I was tired of being pregnant. On top of that, I was a few days overdue. The decision was made to induce. I asked the doctor; he gave a pending date if I did not deliver before the date given and I was in total agreement. The day came when it was time to deliver, and I did just that. I was induced, but there was very little response after multiple hours of Pitocin and pain. I was told that her heart rate was dropping, and an emergency cesarean would be needed. I was scared. I did not know what to expect, because this had never been a part of the plan. I had to take myself out of the situation mentally to keep from upsetting myself in any way. I remembered asking the doctor, "Is it true that I will never have a flat stomach again?" He laughed and said that it is not true. We both chuckled a bit and off to delivery we went. At that point, the mood was lightened, and I was ready to get the show on the road. I was prepped, put to sleep, and woke up with a beautiful baby girl. I was even more determined, eager, and ready to jump start things where I left off. I had to regain my Nike mindset: "Just do it."

Life's Nugget

Never underestimate what
others see in you.

Life's Nugget

If your vision is not clear as it relates
to your future, hold on to the
potential that others see within you
until you can identify the same.

Can you identify why you are stuck and what is the first step to move beyond your reasons (i.e., fears, insecurities, comfortabilities, etc.)?

What has been your most intimidating moment and how did you move forward with your plan despite how you felt?

How have you handled situations that were unplanned and unexpected while trying to reach a goal?

____

____

____

____

What traumatic event have you experienced and how has it helped you with life decisions?

____

____

____

____

CHAPTER SEVEN

You Determine the Outcome

Sometimes it is the very thing that is unexpected that causes you to push even harder. To know that the game had changed from one mouth to feed to two. The reality of making things happen was even more important to me now more than ever. Six weeks had passed, and I returned to work. Several months later I re-enrolled at Indiana University Northwest. This time it was different, with a more intense reason and purpose to complete the program. I was so determined that I took 19 credit hours each semester. I felt like I was trying to regain time that I had lost. It was exhausting yet rewarding because I knew just how determined I was to complete this phase in my life. Going to school after having children was not easy, but it gave it more meaning. It was not easy, with studying, deadlines, papers, exams, and the list went on and on, but I was ready to withstand whatever was needed to make things happen.

At the time, the church I attended was directly up the street from school. I attended prayer on my lunch hour faithfully because the thought of failing was not an option. I had to pull on everything I knew to do to get me through the program. Studying was a must for me. I can recall recording every lecture and writing everything down word by word. Waking up in the wee hours of the morning to read, write papers, study, practice presentations, etc. was a routine. The multiple classes that I decided to take were hectic but manageable. The midnight shift became my best friend. There was already internal pressure felt from the number of credit hours I was taking, but my goal was to complete the program. I had a lot on my plate, but I was determined to eat it all.

The A/P (anatomy and physiology) professor did not make it any better. His introduction from day one was intimidating. There were no smiles or greetings, just warnings, expectations, and observations. I called it "The reality eye opener." The class was held in an auditorium. The professor was an older gentleman who was approximately 6'8", wore glasses and demanded attention as he would stand on the stage and walk back and forth, not having to say a word. He made it perfectly clear from the very first day that many of us would not survive his class. "Look around the room," he said. "More than half of you will not pass this class. If you are working, quit your jobs. You will not have a life while taking this class." I thought, *OMG who says that? What in the hell have I gotten myself into?* This made me feel even worse. The intimidation went through the roof. It felt like there was a siren going off in my head. Talking about an instant headache! My mouth was extremely dry, and my heart was pounding so fast that I thought it was going to jump out of my chest. I believed in that moment I was having a true scare attack; it was way beyond anxiety and panic alone. I had to leave the room, catch my breath, and drink some water. The moment had come when I had to use what I had been taught. Pastor Charles Jones had equipped me with a good foundation and the essential tools that I was able to use every step of the way. I can recall us having a conversation in which he said, "Daughter, sometimes you have to know how to encourage yourself." That moment had arrived. I looked in that mirror and said to myself, "Deb, you can do this. You will finish. That message was not for you. Pick yourself up and know that you got this." I got myself together. Like they say, I pulled my bootstraps up, put my big girl panties on and said, "Okay girl, let's do this."

I went back into the room, took my seat, and was determined not to become one of the statistics that he spoke about. It was not easy, but I never had to experience the outcome that was so clearly, precisely, and confidently announced to an auditorium full of individuals with a goal to pass his class and complete whatever program they enrolled in. The professor was 100% correct by the end of the semester. Over half of the students that started with me had failed the class. He called it just as it occurred. I saw the devastation on some of the students' faces as they saw their score from the final exam. It was a sad day for many, and my instructor made it perfectly clear on day one what the outcome was going to be. He was immune to it, because he saw the same thing every semester. I had initially planned to get my associates degree, but the more I thought about it, the more I realized I should just keep going. I did just that. My counselors and nursing instructors were very helpful. I was informed of the LPN to BSN accelerated program. They spoke and I listened. I thought to myself, *Hey, why not?* They were always there to listen and assist as needed. I remember when I would walk to their offices or the classroom, I would take time to look at the pictures on the walls of the previous nurse graduates and say to myself, "One day it's going to be me up there." That image of me being on the wall of graduates stayed fresh in my mind. It was an addition to the motivation processes that I was already pulling on. Working, school, kids, wife, life all balled up in one. This was when I got it: valid excuses can always be made, but they can limit, decrease, or tear down what is trying to be established or built by the individual that makes them.

By this time, the hospital where I was working had an all-staff meeting. It was announced that the hospital was going to close. Mercy Hospital had experienced financial hardships, and despite some of the physicians banding to-gether to try to save it, their attempts were unsuccessful. It was a very sad day when the patients had to be transferred and the hospital was empty. The building was so silent that you could hear a pin drop. There were many tears shed and a lot of goodbyes being said. The hospital had such an incredible family-like environment. It seemed that no matter what the needs were, someone was always available to assist. Many individuals walked away with a heavy heart. I take my hat off and applaud the physicians that were in the forefront of trying to do everything possible to save the hospital from sinking. They did not go down without a good fight. I can recall the late Dr. Nwabara saying to me, "We are trying and hoping it all will work out." But I knew in that moment that it was just a matter of time. The look he had on his face said it all. As I walked out of the building on my last day, I stood in the parking lot and was even more determined to stay focused and finish what I had started. The enjoyment, knowledge, and experiences that I gained from working at Mercy Hospital and having clinical there was never to be forgotten, but to be built upon. It was at another crossroad that I have come to learn that this is what life is all about.

I had to work, but I also needed to finish school. I decided not to be tied down by a schedule, so I worked for an agency instead. In the beginning it was great. I was able to work without any real obligations to a particular establishment. I chose when, where and what shift I wanted to work. I was assigned to hospital and nursing homes that had staffing needs. In many cases I had a brief orientation, and the expectation was for me to be able to carry out the assignments given without much assistance. Many times, the places where I would go would give me the worst assignments – the ones that no one wanted to work due to various reasons, such as a heavy caseload, multiple behaviors, a huge medication pass that included multiple IVs, and the majority of the patients requiring total assist (meaning you had to do everything for them) just to name a few. I never complained. I was taught and mentored by some amazing individuals. I was not afraid of hard work. I was no stranger to bathing, showering, passing meds, incontinent care, speaking with families, doing wound care, and other skilled bedside procedures. I never had the luxury of having a wound care nurse or team. I was accustomed to providing that one-on-one care. Oh yeah, several assignments required bedside nursing, meaning you were the nurse and the aide. That was what I called being responsible for all duties that involved the whole patient to promote wellness. During several assignments that I would go on, the staff and other management personnel would attempt to hire me. I always refused, because I liked the idea of not being fully committed at the time. The plan was to leave an impression so employment could be steady and consistent. Like any good thing, my time ran out. The facilities were hiring, and I noticed my shifts began to be canceled more and more. Thankfully, I had made it through the first two years of the program which allowed me to obtain an Associate's while completing my Baccalaureate degree. I had made plans to take off the summer and return in the fall. It was not easy, but it was worth it all. As an LPN (licensed practical nurse), I learned what to do. As an RN (registered nurse), I was learning the theory and management as to the why we do what we do as a nurse. I was ready to explore other phases of nursing because I was still on the road to find my niche.

I heard a lot about home health and the flexibility that it would give. As the agency assignments decreased, I was employed working for a home health agency. To begin with, I enjoyed it. It was very flexible. I scheduled my time around my patient. Some visits I had to make more than once in a day because they left and did not inform me. There was an experience I had that I will never forget. I had a very young female patient who I was assigned to who required extensive wound care. She was a gunshot victim and required dressing changes to the back of both her legs, buttock, hips and back. She lived in a housing project that had only one way in and one way out. When I would go into the home, I never felt 100% secure for some reason. She had a boyfriend who would always be there when I arrived, and on a few occasions a few of his friends would be there as well. Her mother would always sit in a living room chair as if she were safeguarding something. She would look at me and speak, pointing to the back room where her daughter was. I would follow her lead, and my patient was always welcoming and excited to see me. There were a few occasions when the home would be very dim, and I would have to ask them to turn on lights before I would enter the home. The atmosphere was odd. I could not explain it, but I knew it did not feel right. I expressed this to my director of nursing. She did not give me much reassurance, other than mentioning that the home had been checked out prior to picking up the client and all was well. Something was off about this and I felt it. I just could not put my finger on it right away. I expressed that I wanted to have my assignment changed because I felt so uncomfortable. My director refused to reassign me but stated that she was going to accompany me on my next visit. I agreed, but I was still unsure about it. I was trying not to ruffle any feathers. The conversation took place at the end of the day on a Friday. I was not scheduled to see the patient until that following Monday at approximately 11:00 am. Given how uncomfortable I felt about going back, it was all I could think about over that weekend. I was nervous and felt a very eerie feeling. There was a pit in my stomach as I watched each hour pass by. On Monday morning at approximately 7:30 am, my patient's mother called me. I was shocked! She had never called me in the past. I instantly thought something was wrong – either my patient was in the hospital or worse. As she said who she was, I was curious and yet concerned as to why she was calling. I was nowhere near prepared for what she was about to say to me. She warned me not to come back to the home again. I asked if everything was okay. She then informed me that she overheard her daughter's boyfriend and some of his friends discuss how they were planning on raping me on my next visit. I was shocked and extremely disturbed about what she said to me. She made it clear that they would do it. She said she was sorry but did not want me to get hurt. I thanked her and told her I was greatly appreciative that she informed me of their plan. I immediately informed my director and was extremely disturbed by her response. She said the mother must be upset with the daughter and did not want anyone giving her care. I thought to myself, *Is she serious?* Did she not hear what I said on Friday? Did she not hear me say that I had an eerie feeling when I would enter that house? Despite what my director thought, I viewed it as my guardian angel looking out for me. That was the moment when I understood that if I do not speak up for myself no one is going to do it for me. I had never abruptly quit a job throughout my entire career, but this was one of those moments where I had to do what I had to do. I had no regrets! Let me see my life versus a paycheck? There is no comparison. My director was adamant about me making the 11:00 am visit as planned. I was not going to stick around to find out whether the mother's warning was true or not. I was convinced, regardless of the theory my director gave. My days of home health were over. I reiterated what the mother informed me of, and made it clear that I was not going back there. I had to be the expert of my own life. I never looked back, and I never desired to. After that experience I took off for a while. It was upsetting and frightening to think about what could have happened. To know that the simple act of listening and taking heed to what was said is what could have changed the trajectory of my life. It is something for me to be thankful for. Who knows how different an ending that story could have had if I did not stand up for myself? I was glad that I had enough boldness and common sense to make a wise decision. I was being influenced to do something that was not in my best interest. It was a situation that did not call for much thinking on my part. I was clear. I thought it was sad that the significance of what was reported was not taken seriously or as a threat. It was time to move on.

School had started again, and this was my chance to bring things together to prepare myself for the hectic schedule that I signed up for. I focused on school for several months before I returned to work. I had missed the hospital and enjoyed working in that environment, so I decided to go back into that setting. I applied at Methodist Hospital north campus and got a job working on the Cardiac IMCU unit. I gained even more experience and skills, from telemetry monitoring, reading cardiac strips, mixing and administering specific medications, and assisting the physician with bedside procedure. It was exciting to see myself growing. I would often do a self-check just to gauge my knowledge and skillset to verify that it was moving in the right direction. Ms. Bernard was the director of the unit. She was very intelligent, stern and expected her unit to run smoothly. The nurses made sure of that. The unit was very busy. I would often say that there were not enough hours in the day. I worked 7-3 and 3-11. If there was a call-off, someone had to stay if there was no replacement. We all would rotate based on seniority. Millie was a classmate that was hired at the same time on the same unit that I was. So, you guessed it, we were at the bottom of the totem pole, and yes, we were stuck to cover on several occasions. Ms. Bernard worked with our school schedules, but she explained that there was nothing she could do if there was a call-off. School, kids, studying, etc., etc., etc. I can recall one night I worked the 3–11 shift and was mandated to work 11–7. I had gotten no sleep. The night before, my youngest daughter had not been feeling well and I had to study for a test. I was already exhausted, tired, miserable, and sleepy for my shift. I barely made it, so when I was told I had to stay for the 11–7 shift I had an instant headache. I had to do something, and fast. I was absolutely no good. My body was completely worn out.

Despite the love I had for the unit, I had to ultimately look out for me. I set up a meeting with the director and expressed to her that the shifts and hours were causing a strain on my physical wellbeing. I decreased my shifts to twice a week, excluding any of my school days. I decided to pick up some additional time at a nursing home. I figured I knew the expectations and it would make up for the days that I was giving up at the hospital without the additional demands. I applied at Timberview Nursing Home and was hired to work on the north unit. I was a floor nurse and was pulled to assist on special projects and processes as they related to system management and regulatory compliance. I made it clear that I did not mind assisting. I did not want to be responsible for a management role without the capability of being able to give the time needed to effectively meet the expectations. My focus was to finish school. As time drew closer for me to graduate, I noticed that I began to gravitate toward long-term care. There was an unspoken internal gratification that I had in these contexts. The director at the time was very sharp with years of experience. She would talk about the regulations as if she wrote them herself. She would do rounds and look at the clinical records to make sure follow-up was done. She would ask questions that were thought-provoking and would assist the nurses or the aide with the answer. Her goal was to make sure they had a good understanding and knew the important questions they should be asking as they were getting reports. To watch her do rounds with wound care and periodically dress wounds was highly impressive. She worked very well with everyone. Doris was the gastrointestinal nurse practitioner (GI NP) who would come to the building often, make rounds on her assigned residents and give orders. I would draw on her often for information and explanations regarding some of the orders that she would give. I recalled saying to her, "One day I'm going to be an NP." She would always say to let her know if I ever needed any help. I was interested in learning, building, and developing with the goal of mastering as much as I could to increase my knowledge base. I noticed how nurse leadership had their own individual way of doing things. I was able to identify the different methods individuals used to get to the goal, which was the care of the resident. This was something that got a spark out of me. It was exciting to watch, and fulfilling to be a part of a team that respected my focus on school and understood that I could assist on special assignments without taking a leadership position.

I eventually resigned from the hospital. The decision was not an easy one, because the wealth of learning and knowledge that I obtained, not mentioning the ladies that I worked with, were incredible. I resigned shortly before obtaining my BSN (Bachelor of Science of Nursing). I had made up my mind to work full-time in the nursing home despite the fact that the hospital offered to pay me more. I admired how the director of nursing worked and her style of doing things. She was fair, professional, and knowledgeable. Who could have asked for more? I knew that if I studied under her and learned as much as she knew, the sky would be the limit for me one day. She had an open-door policy and always made herself available despite her own workload. It was the qualities and characteristics that I saw in her that made my decision to choose long-term care easier.

Graduation had finally come. It was a major accomplishment knowing that my motivating force was my girls. The hard work and sacrifices finally paid off. I can recall the times when I wanted to throw in the towel. It is part of the human experience that I am sure many can relate. You would have to fill in your own blank as it relates to your situation. Just remember: your decisions, your moves, your action, your reactions, your motives, your motivation, your goals, and your outcomes depend on the tenacity you have within you to make things happen.

Life Lesson

A valid excuse can always be made, but know that it can limit, decrease, or tear down what is trying to be established or built by the individual that is making them.

Life Lesson

Do not be influenced by someone's
opinion that can cause unwanted serious
or negative results because they choose
to ignore the obvious warning signs given.
Be careful who has your ear because it can
cost you more than you are willing to pay.

Life Lesson

All progress made toward a goal regardless of the size are steps needed to get to the bigger picture. Do not throw in the towel and give up!

Explain a time when you had to stand up for yourself regardless of what someone in authority wanted you to do.

____

____

____

____

Have you ever had anyone try to influence a decision that you did not agree with? What was it and what was the outcome? Include what it possibly could have been if you would have listened to them.

____

____

____

____

What situation have you experienced that you knew a guardian angel showed up just in time for you?

____

____

____

____

Explain the feeling you had when you completed a goal that you set out to do despite the timeframe that it was finished in.

____

____

____

____

Your Building Capacity Is the True Reflection of Leadership

The time had come for me to build on all that I had gained throughout the years and add to it. The relief of being done with school was a milestone within itself. Things were coming together. I was able to step back and see the building blocks stack up. I was working in an environment that I enjoyed, with an individual that I respected highly and learned a great deal from, as well as finally making the decision to take a leadership role. I was adding to the jar of my life to maximize the capacity to give out what was given to me along the way.

I became the supervisor of the north unit. My director had no issues with sharing her knowledge in anyway. She went above and beyond her duty as a director of nursing. As time went on, like life, things changed. The director of nursing received another job offer that required her to move. I noticed change was inevitable and sometimes even good things must come to an end. I hated that she was leaving but I understood. She was very thorough with me and reviewed systems that I had never been exposed to. It was as if she was orientating me to her role. I was nowhere near ready for that. On her last day she reassured me and said, "You are going to be great!" It was comforting yet sad at the same time. Her replacement came and the assistant director of nursing (ADON) resigned shortly afterwards. I was asked by the new director to take on the role of ADON. After careful consideration I accepted. It was time for me to pull all that I had learned together to be as successful as possible in my new role. I came to realize that just because you may have a title does not mean that you are doing what is needed to get the job done. The new director's style of management was different than the previous one. She was not hands-on. She depended on me to make rounds and report concerns. I found myself going from one end of the facility to the other, following up on complaints or needs, writing reports, auditing, etc. You name it, I found myself doing it.

The facility needed a clinical nurse consultant to assist in the needs of the facility as it related to nursing development and clinical outcome. I welcomed whatever assistance that was being offered. The facility was looking to find someone who had at heart the best interest of the residents and the development of the people who worked there. Gwen was a consultant who had worked in long-term care in other states. She was exactly what the facility needed. I knew her and I was convinced she was the person for the job. I made arrangements for her to meet with the regional. She was exactly what was needed. She came on board and was an excellent addition to the facility. I had the help and support that I could go to, to assist in processes and protocol that needed to be put in place to move the facility forward. I had expressed to her that I was considering quitting. She gave me the best advice without hesitation concerning my future, professionalism, growth, maturing and advancement. She sat me down in the office and gave me these words of wisdom. "Slow down, make time in your day to have a lunch. You must learn how to take a mental break. You will burn yourself out if you do not take time out of your day for you. You must stay in your role – or any leadership role – for at least a year." She said it would help build my resume. I understood that I was growing in knowledge and skillset; now it was time for me to build on paper. She also made me realize that with all the things I was doing it was allowing me to become more efficient. The more she would audit, review, and put systems in place, the more understanding and clarity I gained. I stopped complaining about what I was doing despite not being the person responsible for it. She allowed me to see that the more information I had, the better presentation I would have to give with whatever situation I encountered. This would be proven true in more ways than one.

As time passed, my growth and development continued to progress. The director I worked with did not change. The more she did not do, by default allowed me to become more knowledgeable in areas that I would not have been. I was determined to be efficient in every area that I was exposed to, from reporting, assessing, follow-up, making rounds, educating, auditing, making clinical decisions and much more. It was not often that I would have the office to myself. It was odd: my director was off, and normally I would do follow-ups on the units, but on this day I did them in the office. I received a call that was very unexpected. The caller asked if I was the ADON and I answered, "Yes, I am." She proceeded to say that she was a recruiter and wanted to have an interview set up for a director of nursing position. I was silent for a few seconds because this was my first call from a recruiter. I thought to myself, *Is this normal?* I later found out that it was. I got myself together and a follow-up call was scheduled. I was not sure if I was ready to take on such responsibility. I had conquered the year experience like I was advised, but I thought to myself, *Now what?* I consulted with Gwen, and she advised me to look more into it. I started to think about the mentors I had, the life lessons I learned, the knowledge I gained and the direction of leadership that I was growing in. The more I thought about it the more I was convinced within myself to think, "Why not me?" I had made the decision to move forward after having several conversations and interviewing with the other company. I met with my director and the administrator, and they counter-offered, and asked if I would be the director of nursing there. My director stated that she would go to another facility within the company. I also received a call from one of the owners, Gary Ott, to see what could be done to get me to stay. Despite them offering me more money, the call from the owner, and a promotion, I knew that was not my building to direct. I was flattered, thankful, but I was convinced that my time had come to an end there. It was time for me to take the next steps that were critical to my success. I had no doubt in my mind that this was what I needed to do.

Thirty days later I became the director of nursing at Clark Road Nursing and Rehabilitation. I never desired to be an ADON let alone DON (director of nursing), but I was always opened to explore, develop, and conquer my fears of the unknown. I was very nervous and unsure of my capabilities. I had been exposed to many processes, but I was not sure of what I did not know. I even had a parking space but did not park in it for months. I felt like even though I had the position, I did not have the position. Meaning I may have had the title, but I was not convinced that I knew enough to get the expected results. I took things one day at a time. I studied the policies and procedures. I incorporated processes that I knew. I consistently met with the nursing team. I held individuals accountable. I made rounds and met with each resident. I poured into others and educated them as much as possible. I was determined to learn the residents' first and last names. I met with the team members to review and discuss expectations. The nurse management team complimented the flow of the clinical system well. They carried out assignments and follow-ups on pertinent information that was related to the residents' care. We held meetings to ensure the residents were properly cared for and processes were being followed. Jessie, Surney, Tina, Ava, Tara, and Michelene were some of the managers that assisted in processes that were needed to move the building forward. I had a clear understanding that leadership flowed from the top and the climate of the facility would be set by the gauge the leadership temperature was on. I believed that it was important to immediately confront offenses, misunderstandings, or negative perceptions within leadership to prevent the focus from being lost. The goal was to have good clinical outcomes, which is much easier to do when the cancer of discord has not fumigated the atmosphere. I can truly say that these women took their positions seriously, were clear on their roles and were able to produce what was expected without hesitation. They were instrumental in allowing me to develop in my role as a DON. I was able to see things moving in the right direction, processes put in place, audits conducted, effective follow-up and the staff in sync with the protocols implemented. I had to take a moment to realize that a lot of what I thought I was lacking was already in me. It was just a matter of me recognizing it. I had built up enough tenacity to eventually park in the space that was assigned to me. I finally got it: it was not about the parking space; it was about me understanding what I was called to do in that time of my life and own it. I gained what I needed and had to discover that I was carrying it within me all along. It was truly an awakening, because all I needed to do was to trust what I knew and continue to be open to learn more. It was an amazing discovery that I tapped into.

I worked with several administrators during my tenure. Eric Simon was one of them that I worked with at Clark Road. Periodically a friend of his named Michael would come to the facility to visit. He stood approximately 5'7", had dark black hair, a medium build, with a very distinctive voice. The building overall was running well clinically. He would always ask me to come work for him where he was the administrator-in-training at a sister facility. I would always say that I was not leaving, and he would respond by saying, "One day you are going to work for me." I would always respond with a smile and say, "Okay." Little did I know how significant those words would be. One thing about the healthcare industry is that you never know when you will bump into someone again on your professional journey. Life has a way of making you go in a complete circle sometimes, seeing those very people who you started with or met along the way. The saying is true: "Your first impression may be the only one you get to make." Remember to always strive to be the best version of you. You never know when it may count. Several years passed and I would often think about Doris the

NP from my previous employer. She was a hard worker and had the residents' best interest at heart. I appreciated the time she would take out with others to explain her findings or her methods to assist in problem solving. She set a good example and was very motivating to watch in action.

The more I would reminisce about the experiences I had with her, the more I thought about returning to school. It did not take me long to decide. I remembered what I had said several years prior concerning me going back to become a nurse practitioner. I enrolled at Purdue University after discovering the program worked around my schedule. I was not in a rush and my current employer offered tuition reimbursement. All I had to do was pass the classes and they reimbursed me at 100%. I was approached by my employer on several occasions to become an administrator while I was in school. I was not interested, and again my focus was to make sure the building was running appropriately, and that I finished the program. It is easy to pile your plate full and not get anything properly eaten or digested. I understood that I had to make the main thing, the main thing. My consultant was very supportive. What I appreciated was that she never came to run the building. She gave me the ability to utilize my abilities, autonomy, and structure to move the building forward. Her focus was always to support and make sure I had what I needed to be successful. She was approachable and consistent. She would give guidance as needed. Her visits would consist of multiple focuses, which included but were not limited to giving her updates, reviewing charts, staffing, or auditing just to name a few. There were times when she would come to the facility just to make sure I was okay. She would mention how she wanted to become the risk management nurse and wanted me to become a nurse consultant. I declined every time she asked. I had to remind her that, until I had completed school, I would not take on a new role. She understood but she kept it fresh on my mind. I was excited about going back. Things had changed as it related to my situation, growth, mindset, role, professionalism, and maturity. My girls were older. I had more confidence and boldness. I had experience under my belt, and I was comfortable in my role.

During the program I started having some mild symptoms: an occasional upset stomach, slight nausea in the mornings, I just was not feeling well. I could not explain what I was feeling, but it was different. I had to take a class in Washington, DC, but the day before I was scheduled to leave my ADON had a beautiful basket on my desk and was wishing me a safe trip. Within the basket was a blue and white box. I recalled seeing the negative and positive sign. I immediately looked at her and she said, "We need to get to the bottom of why you haven't been yourself. It may explain why you are not feeling well." I had chalked it up to stress, but little did I know stress came with two legs, two arms, a head, and a complete body. To my surprise I was pregnant. I had never considered that in a thousand years. I began to think to myself, *Every time I decide to go to school, I get pregnant.* It was not a laughing matter at that time. This child would be 14 and 11 years younger than my other two little ladies respectively. I was in disbelief for a long time. Once it was identified why I was not feeling well, I did not have any further symptoms. I carried throughout the entire program. I must say that I became a believer very quickly: one month after graduating from the program I gave birth to my beautiful daughter. I took some time off and when I returned to work things were moving. I did the majority of my clinicals for my practitioner program with the medical director. Arrangements were made for me to work with him once I graduated in conjunction with my position as a DON. It worked out great. I would run the office for several days and make rounds on residents. My roles were different in the two settings, but the one thing that brought them both together was having the skillset to properly assess, have good critical thinking skills, and develop or evaluate the treatment plan that was implemented. I worked in a family practice setting, so my patients included prenatal wellness checks, pediatrics to geriatrics. I was always very fond of my geriatric patients. They always brought a touch of wisdom or energy that brightened the day. I discovered early on that I enjoyed learning, and the field of healthcare gave me just that.

I eventually took on the request to become a nurse consultant for the company. My consultant's name was Stephanie. She took the time to train me and was always open to answer any questions that I may have had. What I quickly realized was that facilities can be under one umbrella but function very differently. The approach for one building was not necessarily the approach that could be used for another. Every building had their own style and way of doing things. In whatever facility I was assigned to, I would do an observational assessment. The plan was to determine what was working and change what was not. The overall goal was to always identify the team players to formulate a plan that could be implemented and executed. I understood that buy-in and being approachable were key elements in attempting to change dynamics or implement systems. People needed to trust in what I was doing and believe I had the ability to make change happen.

After working as a consultant for less than a year I was asked by the owner (Mr. Rowthner) to take on a facility that was having some difficulties and was scheduled to close if citations were not cleared and the conditions did not improve. I reviewed the citations and a plan was implemented. I met with the administrator and took on the responsibility. I met with the team and explained the task that was ahead of us. It was not going to be easy, but I was convinced that it was possible. Patricia (aka Pat) was one of the managers that worked with me day and night to monitor and assess the plans that were implemented. I was strategic with the follow-up that was needed as well as the education. I ensured that the staff clearly understood what was needed to move the facility forward. I never turned away from a call, regardless of the time. I gave the facility the support that was needed to make effective change happen. The goal was to get everyone on the same page to steer the ship (facility) in the same direction. All-hands-on deck was the game plan to make it happen.

Change was happening and the shift was clearly seen. The return visit was made by the state to evaluate the plan and the changes that were made. The visit was a success! The facility did not close, and the conditions improved. It was a victory to be celebrated, and it goes without saying that rest was well deserved. Even though it took a lot of energy, effort, and time, it paid off in the long run. What I know for sure was that whenever a team comes together with a common goal there is nothing they will not be able to do. Leadership flows from the top down: effective leader, effective team; weak leader, weak team. After several years of service and gaining much experience as a consultant and a director I made the decision to move on to pursue my practitioner career full-time. I was continuing my journey of building capacity. I realized that the responsibility, accountability, and the marketability of who I was becoming and evolving into was setting a precedent within a profession that had become my passion.

Life Lesson

Effective leadership is determined by
the buy-in of the plan that has been
implemented, evaluated, and executed by
those who are following.

Life Lesson

Take advantage when you are exposed to new areas despite someone else being responsible for it. You never know if it is a set-up for your next level of advancement.

Life Lesson

It takes a team moving in the same
direction to get to the desired destination.

Have you ever had to complete assignments that were not your responsibility? If you have, what was it and what was the outcome you experienced from it?

Who has been a positive influence in your life? Explain how they influenced you.

What strategies have you used to bring structure to a situation that you have been involved or in charge of?

____

____

____

____

What experience have you had that caused you to be in denial about a situation? How and what timeframe did it take you to come to reality?

____

____

____

____

What has been the most challenging time that you have faced that required you to put forth additional time and effort to get a specific outcome?

____

____

____

____

Compartmentalize What Is Important

Taking the time to separate each aspect of your life is needed to reflect and evaluate where you have been, where you are going, and whether you are satisfied with where you are. This is something that I often did because my ultimate goal was to be a better version of myself. I had to take those critical times in my life and separate what was important from what was very important, and then what was the priority. As I developed and took on new roles, I realized that every mentor, situation, and experience – good, bad, and ugly – was a product of my growth and development. I had gained not just an understanding of the profession but also the importance of being professional. As I was introduced to new challenges, I realized that each developmental stage of my growth and learning was tapped into. I realized that, while the areas that I worked in were different, the bottom line was that the patients were the priority. So, despite the number of letters behind my name, I never lost sight of my initial orientation, which was the care of the patient. As I worked full-time in the office, it was never anything for me to assist the geriatric patient who needed help. I had friends who had loved ones who were bed-ridden and would ask me to stop by to orient them as to how to provide care, especially when home health was delayed or not initiated for whatever reason. It was rewarding to educate them and walk them through how to turn, reposition, clean, bathe, feed and provide an assessment. I understood that the more knowledge they had concerning their loved one's disease process and skin breakdown prevention, the less likely it was that I would have to treat them in the office.

I eventually transitioned to another family practice office that had a huge clientele. Many mornings the office would be full before I arrived. The pace was nonstop, from the time the doors opened to closing. It seemed as if there was not a disease process that I did not encounter or treat. The experience was very enlightening. What I noticed was that I would encounter inspiring nurses who were having difficulties passing their exams. I had taken time previously to assist an individual by the name of Niki, who had been working as a certified nursing assistant for several years. She had completed the nursing program ten years prior and had been working as an aide even longer. She explained to me how the challenges of life held her back from passing the required state exam or having the desire to even study for it. Niki had experienced some serious challenges, including the death of a loved one, imprisonment of another and illness. She explained how she could not focus and even though she had a desire to become a nurse, her will to do it had been tarnished. Her situation weighed heavy on me. I decided to take on the task and helped her reach her goal. I made it very clear that as long as she worked around my schedule and was ready to meet whenever I had the availability, without formulating any excuses or negativity, I assured her that she would pass. I had never seen anyone as motivated. I had to restructure the negative thinking into positive thinking. The goal was to get her to prioritize what she needed to do to obtain the prize. There were creative assignments given so she could visualize herself as a nurse. I had her sign her name numerous times as if she had passed her boards and was a nurse. My goal was to make sure she had the understanding and the clarity on prioritizing, disease processes, critical thinking, and a list of other needed criteria to pass the exam. I often explained to her, "If you can understand the why, it will take you through the processes." It was not just study sessions; it was self-building sessions as well. All I had to keep on the forefront of her mind was, "Why not you?" I advised her that when she was ready to take the exam, she was not to tell anyone, including me. I needed her to stay focused to reduce her anxiety as much as possible. Everything that could have been reviewed was. She was able to answer questions regardless of how they were formulated. I knew she was ready and able to stand on her own two feet. After several months of intense studying, she achieved her goal, and she became a licensed practical nurse (LPN). The overwhelming joy she experienced was breathtaking. Her thanks were countless, her joy was infectious. I asked her in return to honor two requests—one, to give back to help someone else along the way, and two, to be the best nurse she could be. She obliged without hesitation.

Having that experience, along with others, including the multiple inspiring nurses that I met, caused me to launch my business, D. Givens Consulting and Health Education. I have assisted an exceeding number of nursing students with obtaining their license. To have the opportunity to assist someone else on their journey was an excellent way for me to give back and point someone in the right direction toward their road to success. It is a rewarding feeling to know that you have assisted in someone's life when they were on the brink of throwing in the towel. I enjoyed my role as an NP as well as the educational support that I was providing the students. I cannot explain it, but it came to a point that I sought out change as it related to working in the office.

One day at approximately 3:30 am I was searching the internet to see what jobs were being featured. I happened to come across an organization that needed a regional nurse to oversee several buildings. I thought to myself that this seemed to be very interesting. As I read the job description, I thought to myself, *I can do this,* so I submitted my resume. I must admit I did have three concerns. The job was in Chicago, Illinois, so it would be far from where I was familiar with. I also knew that the traffic in Chicago is bad, and that the city's drivers' have a bad reputation. To my surprise, between 6:30 and 7:00 am the next morning I received a call from a gentleman with a very distinguished yet familiar voice. "May I speak to Debra Givens?" he asked.

"This is she," I replied.

"Do you know who this is?"

It took me a few seconds, then it dawned on me who I was speaking to. It was the administrator-in-training who would come to my building years prior and ask me to come work for him. I was shocked and immediately remembered him saying to me, "One day you are going to work for me." My response to that comment was always, "Okay." I guess my okay was coming to fruition. I would not have ever guessed that we would have crossed paths years later, but we did. The conversation went on and he asked what I did that morning. It was then that I realized I must have sent my application to a company that he was affiliated with. I laughed and said, "You have to be kidding." I told him that I sent my resume for a regional position.

He then laughed and said, "It's my company. When can you start?"

I had an interview with two of his key personnel and a month and a half later I took on the role. That was the timeframe it took me to conquer my fears of driving in the Illinois traffic. I canceled my start date twice due to my driving fears. I eventually got to the point that I was able to drive from one part of Illinois to another without any hesitation. I experienced organizational and personal growth during my tenure.

I believe that continual evolving should be the internal expectation of any individual regardless of the setting they are in. The job had a lot of demands due to the multiple facilities for which I was responsible. The expectations were clearly spelled out and others were learned along the way. Some of the expectations were to be accountable, take responsibility, be proactive, understand system management, provide education, and have positive outcomes. The name of the game was results, results, results. I enjoyed meetings with the team when resolutions to specific issues where addressed and plans were executed. I would listen to the owner during our meetings and his ideas and perceptions of the industry, problem solving and anything else that required non-box theory thinking. I learned that another responsibility was to sit as the clinical leader within the facilities when there were vacancies. I can recall during my first year and a half I sat in a facility and assumed the role of the director in a building that we had taken over. There were a lot of challenges and a lot of bad habits that the staff had acquired throughout the years. My job was to interrupt the patterns and implement systems, processes, and procedures via education and training.

There was not any nurse manager, and I had the weight of trying to work out how to make it all come together. What I quickly learned was that everything cannot always be controlled, but the expectation was that you had control over of it. I remember thinking, "How do I wrap my head around that concept and get the intended results?" I felt myself spinning my wheels because of the way the staff was accustomed to doing things. The resistance and the challenge were that much greater. I had gotten to the point that I wanted to give up. I began to do what many nurses have as weaknesses, but do not always realize it, and that is to do things themselves because then we know things are done. I knew this was not good but the lack of clinical support and the staff resistance to change was a constant fight that I was not accustomed to. I noticed that I was burning myself out. I had decided to turn in my resignation and when I did, it was handed right back to me. I had a sit down right in that moment with the same person who said where I would be working years earlier. He said, "I don't need you to do the work, I need you to put the knowledge that you have in them." It was as if he had me look inside myself and destroy the box that I created concerning the possibility of things not improving. He also said, "I need you to get out of the building at a reasonable time daily." From that day forward, I received a call daily to go home at 4:00 pm. It was a gesture that I often think about to this day. An intervention was needed, and it was given just in time. With time, the pieces started coming together. Two nurses stepped up to the plate to assist me. Vernedia and Tammy jumped in and supported every action that was put in place. They had worked for the company and were the clinical support I needed to assist to gain clinical compliance. Taking on a challenge is always manageable when you have the tools needed to make things happen. It was not easy, but the support that was given made the processes that were needed successful. That taught me not to get caught up in what is occurring but to take a moment and assess the situation as best as possible and execute a plan that will evoke change and prevent personal burnout. Things were moving along and were going well.

A few years later life happened. I found myself trying to balance work, kids and responsibilities while going through a divorce. I was determined that despite what I was experiencing I was not going to let my personal impact my professional. I had to make a conscious decision that I walked through this stage of my life without my employment being affected by it. I missed one day, and no one knew what I was going through. It was not easy, but it was necessary. Once I got over that time in my life, I was determined to be even more purposeful than I was previously. Purposeful in my evolvement, my mindset, my capabilities and everything else that exemplified a leader, not just in my professional role but in my personal one as well. As the years progressed, I was being stretched even more in my thinking and my ability to problem solve, support, respond, multi-task, educate, follow-up, audit, survey prep, think critically, plan and much, much more. I had sat in most of our building due to vacancies to lead the team in having positive clinical outcomes. There was a time that I began to feel that I was the go-to person if there was a need in a building for clinical leadership. I did not mind much, because the buildings that I would cover outside of mine were my VP's. I understood the workload she had on her plate. Illinois was different than Indiana, but I felt like I had the best of both worlds. I worked with some amazing individuals. They were some of the hardest working consultants that I had ever met. They understood teamwork, and regardless of the problems, they were always willing to jump in and assist. After several years of being in my role I would often think about how I was able to adapt to another way of thinking and get the results desired.

I recall one day I was en route to one of the facilities and I received a call from my COO. It was unusual for her to call, but this call was different. The position of vice president of clinical services was open, and she asked me to consider taking it. I was flattered and unsure at the same time. I was comfortable in the role I was in and I wanted to make sure it would not take more time than I was giving. I paused for a minute and expressed to her how I felt, and asked if I could think about it. I recalled having conversations with my previous VP Donna who would often say to me, "You can do my job." I never knew why she would say that, because I never expressed that I wanted to be the VPCS. I later thought maybe she just wanted me to know. I was curious to know what the job entailed before I committed. I had the opportunity to speak to the chief nurse officer (CNO) who explained the job description and what her expectations were. After having that conversation, I felt ready and took on the new role. I would meet with multiple disciplines and outside consultant teams to ensure that the objectives were being met. My goal was to build the relationships and connect the dots that had been disconnected to have better outcomes. Education would consistently be given to enhance the knowledge base of the clinical leader to assist in the development of their teams. I also would visit the facilities to make sure compliance was being met. I later was informed that the CNO was no longer with us. My COO stepped in to support as needed. I routinely met with her to review facilities and any other concerns or issues that may have arisen. Things were always busy with something needing to be done. I understood the responsibility and the task that I had taken on. I was dedicated and committed, with the desire to have the best exemplified via resident care, staff development, system development and facility outcomes. Tami T., one of the VPs of another area, would always check in on me to make sure things were going okay and give advice that was always helpful. The consultant team did what was needed so the facilities felt supported. The goal was that they did not feel alone when they faced a crisis or interruption that required additional assistance.

In the beginning things were moving in the right direction. But in March 2020, all hell broke loose when the pandemic hit, and it turned the world of healthcare into something I had never witnessed in my 28 years of nursing. From the PPE, the constant CDC changes, COVID deaths and illnesses to the universe watching the increase of numbers day by day. It was scary to say the least. I personally lost my grandfather due to COVID and my aunt from complications of COVID. There were countless other staff members who were personally affected by it as well. It was a sad time in healthcare, but the employees continued to show up and do their due diligence to ensure the residents were cared for. There was a time when every available personnel were needed to assist with all aspects of the facility needs. In support of what was needed I scrubbed up and provided direct patient care and whatever else was needed. Despite over time the COVID numbers improving, vaccines being created, and injections being given, the damage was done. Many nurses walked away from the setting to go somewhere less stressful, while others hung their nursing hats up for good. It was the first time the company had to have assistance from an outside agency to assist in residents care. The lack of committed staff, vacancies and other factors played major roles in some of the facility's challenges. What I quickly realized was that this issue was not just one organization's issues, it was throughout the healthcare industry. I found myself filling in the role as the clinical leader in buildings back-to-back to meet the need because clinical leadership was needed. When you are in a position of leadership, that means that at times you may have to fill other critical roles because you do not have the individuals to fill them.

It is ironic how life happens. Things went in one complete circle. The last facility I sat in as the clinical leader had some huge challenges due to multiple factors – some that were avoidable and others that were not. There were system failures and an effective immediate plan needed to be implemented. The time, the sacrifice, the selflessness, and the commitment I had were not just for the company but also for every assignment or role I fulfilled. Even though I was in this facility to get them back on track, I conducted several training sessions with the other facilities' directors because they were new in their buildings. I needed them to get as much guidance as possible so they would know the company's ways of doing things. I gave support and took calls as needed to make sure their facility needs were cared for in conjunction with running a facility. There was a lot that was needed and fast. They were expecting follow-up visits from the state and the goal was to make sure everything was in order. There were missing key clinical positions but there were those who got on the bandwagon and did their due diligence to assist me with the needed elements to put things in place. The facility was cooperative and adhered to the education that was provided. I spent a lot of one-on-one time with the nurses and assisted immediately with any change of conditions to make sure all was being captured. Due to the multiple processes that needed to be put in place, and with the help of the department heads, things were coming together. The staff was understanding and cooperative with the changes that were needed. It was truly a day-by-day process.

I thought about my first time sitting as a director with this company. Time truly brings about change. I pondered on how the last time around I knew exactly what was needed despite not having all the key players. I had my systematic way of doing things that had been proven to work at other times. Regardless of what they were experiencing, I knew that with the diligence and time that was being given all concerns would have been cleared. My tenure with this company was 12 years. I grew with this company and took every lesson to heart. As I reflect on 28 years of serving others, I would not change a thing. Every experience that I have encountered, the good, the bad and the ugly, have equipped me to become the leader that I am today.

Leadership means different things to many people, but to me it entails several key characteristics that I believe are important:

1. Take action and be intentional with decisions that need to be made.

2. Effectively manage conflict.

3. Understand team approach regardless of if it is your idea.

4. Don't just take responsibility when things go well – take it when things don't go as planned.

5. Identify the role you played in a negative outcome.

6. Choose fair treatment over favoritism.

7. Know that saying that you were wrong is not a sign of weakness.

8. Don't take things personal.

9. Admit that you don't know and seek out the answer.

10. Eliminate your ego.

11. Make judgments based on facts, not perceptions.

12. Communicate effectively and respectfully regardless of position.

13. Listen and do not be quick to respond until you fully understand the issue.

14. Empower the team and not your ego.

15. Observe and learn behaviors or practices that are to be encouraged, and those that need to be eliminated.

16. Anticipate when change is needed and make the necessary change.

17. Mirror the behavior you want to see in others: lead by example.

18. Identify and know the strengths and weaknesses of your team.

19. Stay away from gossiping, a sure way trust is quickly lost.

20. Motivate and encourage what you want to see.

21. Never let them see you sweat.

22. Don't be dismissive.

23. Admit you make mistakes.

24. Allow individuals to develop and display their autonomy.

25. Know that your way is not the only way.

26. Apologize when needed.

27. Take control and execute a plan that people can follow.

28. Keep it simple.

29. Educate and verify that individuals understand.

30. Know that a professional approach is the best approach in any situation.

31. Develop your team so everyone is singing the same song.

32. Be mindful of who is in your ear: a hidden agenda or motive could be lurking close by.

33. Rest and know when it's time to take care of you.

Remember: the ultimate goal with anything is to make sure you are becoming a better version of yourself. Take heed to the life lessons that are learned along the way. Never underestimate your potential and always ask, "Why not you?"

Life Lesson

Taking the time to interrupt your agenda for someone who needs help is a selfless act that speaks volumes about your character.

Life Lesson

When you are embarking in new territory take heed and listen before looking for the first exit out. The instructions given may cause you to destroy the box that you did not realize you created.

Life Lesson

Separating the personal from the
professional may not be easy, but it is
necessary to achieve the ultimate goals—
peace and sanity.

What have you done for someone else to assist them on their personal journey to self-improvement?

____

____

____

____

Explain how you approached and completed a specific challenge in your life that initially seemed to be impossible.

____

____

____

____

What changes have affected you personally as it relates to COVID and how are you coping with it?

____

____

____

____

Explain some of the outcomes you have experienced at your place of employment when alternative staff has come to assist?

____

____

____

____

What responsibility have you ever taken on and wanted to know the fine details before accepting? How did it go and what did you learn?

____

____

____

____

NOW WRITE YOUR STORY